# Flabyrinth

### My escape from maximum insecurity prison

## JULES COLL

*Gill Books*

Gill Books
Hume Avenue
Park West
Dublin 12
www.gillbooks.ie

Gill Books is an imprint of M.H. Gill & Co.

© Jules Coll 2016, 2017

978 07171 7906 0

Designed by Síofra Murphy
Printed and bound in Great Britain by Clays Ltd, St Ives plc

Photos on pages 216 and 332 © Ronan Melia Photography

This book is typeset in Garamond.

A CIP catalogue record for this book is available from the
British Library.

5 4 3 2 1

*To my Mr Right, I know you're out there somewhere. Wherever you are, hello from the past. See you in the future xxx*

# Thank you to ...

Conor Nagle, Ruth Mahony, Teresa Daly, Rachel Pierce and all at Gill Books for allowing me to share my story. You have been amazing to work with! (Conor, I look forward to presenting you with your crown very soon!)

Mum and Dad. What can I say? This feels like writing my wedding speech! You are the most wonderful, kind, loving parents a girl could ask for. Thank you for your eternal love and support. And for everything you have done to help me become the happy woman I am today. I am truly grateful and I love you both so much! (And yes, of course, Barry, Gavin and Jennie, I love you too!)

My bestest girlfriends, Donna, Renée and Dawn. Where would I be without my Carrie and two Samanthas?! Thank you for always supporting and encouraging me and making me laugh constantly! I love you all and look forward to annual holidays in Marbs right into our nineties. Spuddies forever! Donna – a special thanks for the past three years of balcony chats as we analysed the lessons to be learned and joined the dots to move forward in life and break those bastard cycles! You're my Dr Phil! Love you!

Andy Pandy, me little posh skanger! What a team we are! Thank you for letting me share your dream because through Damo & Ivor I discovered what I'm meant to be doing in life: writing funny shit! Nobody on the planet makes me laugh more than you! Thanks for all your support, especially for carting me through that feckin' triathlon! Love ya to bits! 'Lickin' my face like a cat!'

Matt Keatley, you're the best personal trainer on the planet. Thank you for teaching me how to work out properly and laugh my ass off as I'm doing it. Exercise has become one of the greatest joys in my life now that I know I'm training effectively under your guidance. Thanks for helping me make the gainz!

Mr Mayilone Arumugasamy, my amazing surgeon. Thank you for saving my life with the intervention of bariatric surgery. I knew I was in the safest of hands with you. Thank you for doing a wonderful job, which enabled me to change my life and health for the better.

And thank you to all of the rest of my friends and family who've loved and supported me throughout my life and weight-loss expedition. And to everyone on social media who's followed my progress and taken the time to send me lovely messages, I really appreciate it.

And some special mentions: Ann and Richard Quirke, Ruth Carter, Eimear Morrissey, all at Parallel Films, Eddie Doyle and Bill Malone. You've all had a big impact on my life and/or career and I truly appreciate your continuous support and belief in me.

# Contents

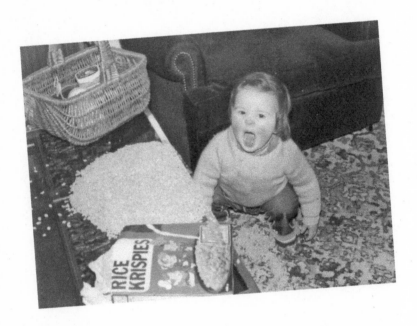

# Introduction: My Escape from Maximum Insecurity Prison

*C*an you imagine how heinous a crime you'd have to commit to warrant being locked up in prison for 15 years? At the tender age of 19, fresh out of school and living the life of Reilly, unbeknownst to me, I had subconsciously sentenced myself to life in the slammer. It would take ten years for me to wake up and realise that I was trapped in prison – a prison of fat. It would take a further five years to realise that I was, in fact, on death row, as I had become morbidly obese.

Before I share with you my story of life in the fat pen and how I did a Shawshank on it and managed to escape, let me introduce myself. My name is Jules I-Didn't-Get-A-Middle-Name Coll, I'm 36 years old, South Dublin born, bred and buttered. What follows in this book is the story of my life explaining how I got fat and eventually slim and how my self-esteem suffered throughout.

I know 99% of people who read this book will be women, so consider right now to be the metaphorical moment that you and I have just met each other in the toilets of a nightclub. We're pissed and crossing our legs in the massive queue for the jacks. I've just admired your handbag and you've told me that it was a fiver in Penney's and I've replied 'No way!' and you're absolutely delighted with yourself and also thinking that you could have told me it cost three grand in Brown Thomas and I would have believed you, so you'll remember that the next time someone admires it. Us girls are all the same. We're a flippin' amazing division of the species: we can give birth, multitask, ask for directions, have multiple orgasms and, I don't care what anyone says, we are great drivers. And yet we're also up to our tits in self-doubt, insecurities and body issues.

So right now I'm throwing my drunken arm around you and letting you know that you're not alone. We are all basket cases crippled by our lack of self-worth and we all spend far too much time listening to and believing the voice inside our head that tells us we're not good enough. I've managed to defeat that voice and I'm sharing my story in the hope that you can do it too. Whether you have a weight issue or even if you've been slim all your life, let's face it who doesn't have insecurities? Even the humanoid robots the Japanese have invented have been programmed with insecurities to make them seem more human!

I've never had a boyfriend in all my days. I'm as single as a microwave meal for one. Reading that you'd probably think 'What the hell is wrong with her? Is she a bunny boiler psycho or an absolute minger?' Have a quick look at my face on the front cover of the book there. What do you reckon? I'd give myself a good six, maybe seven, out of ten after a trip to the hairdressers and with a full face of make-up. I'm alright-looking, I suppose, and I'd like to think that I'm a nice, normal person but that still hasn't enabled me to bag a man and that's because when I was fat, I didn't want any man to come near me. In fact, I was avoiding them at all costs. I would recoil in horror at the thoughts of stripping off and any guy witnessing me in the nip with my extra-large love handles and acres of cellulite. I had more spare tyres than a Kwik Fit garage.

As I write this now, I'm a slim size 10 and do I have a sexy man to make passionate love to my new fit bod?

That would be a no. Which just goes to prove that all this self-esteem bollix really is all tied up in our heads. It's like a big knot of shite. I'm still unravelling mine, but I'm getting there. This is what *Flabyrinth* is all about. While I've achieved so much with my nine-stone weight-loss, and I'm happy to report that the grass is greener on the leaner side, I am still working on myself and manifesting all the things I want. Such is the journey of life, eh? So I decided not to wait until I am 99 and I've learned it all and am on the cusp of my Disney ending before sharing my story from my death bed. I'm only a third of the way through this incarnation and life still has a lot to teach me.

I currently work in TV as a screenwriter and producer for comedy show *Damo & Ivor*. I absolutely love my job. It doesn't feel like work so I know I've found my calling. I've had so many random jobs over the years, including a stint working as a professional Susan Boyle impersonator, and now I can add another string to my bow of bollocks, 'published author'. How fancy! You can't really say that out loud as your job title without sounding like you're at one of the ambassador's receptions in the Ferrero Rocher ad, can you? Luckily I've never been invited to any of his swanky soirées – I would have swiped that big pyramid of chocolate, chucked it into the front seat of my car, wrapped the seatbelt around it to protect it and sped off under the moonlight to have a one-night stand with it.

So how do you go from having a wonderful childhood, being a healthy child, albeit with a serious penchant for sweets but who was slim regardless, to a morbidly obese adult weighing 19 stone, wearing size 22 clothes and feeling like a human version of the Marshmallow Man from *Ghostbusters*? Slowly but surely is the answer. I didn't wake up fat. The weight just crept on over the years, like I was being sculpted by a talentless artist who eventually turned me into a Picasso of poundage. Every so often I'd step on the scales or catch my reflection in the mirror and think 'How the feck did this happen?!' I didn't mean to gain weight, it happened by snaccident.

Did you ever look back at old photos of yourself and wish you were the size you were back then when you thought you were huge? The curse of the fatness is a total bastard. There is no worse feeling than standing at your wardrobe, staring at all your clothes with disgust as you curse them for being so unforgiving and restrictive, thinking, 'I'm so bloated. What can I wear that's comfy?' and blaming your 'meh' mood on your period or the big dinner you just ate, yet all the while knowing that you're looking for the loose clothes because that's all you feckin' fit into. My expedition up Mount Heaviest started off innocently enough after packing on an extra layer of insulation *après* an epic summer of boozing in the Greek islands. I thought I could easily shed the fat once I got home and keep my weight under control. But before I knew it, I was rolling like a chocolate truffle down a mountain of icing sugar and gaining not only momentum but rolls of flab and a bloated pillow face.

I wish there was a way you could donate fat like you can donate blood. Why does food have to be so yummy? Did God really need to give us taste buds? Food can give us so much pleasure and yet so much pain afterwards, if we consume too much of it 'cos it's so feckin' delish. I wish we all had that moderation gene where we could enjoy food, stop eating when we're full and just use food purely as fuel and nourishment. In caveman days it must have been like that. The cavewoman sat in the cave breastfeeding the baby while doodling on the walls because she didn't have a telly to watch. Meanwhile the caveman went out and harpooned a deer to drag home and provide dinner for himself and his family. We live a world away now, surrounded by processed food in pretty packaging, all mass-produced and sold to us with clever marketing that tells us that if we eat it, we will feel incredible, look fantastic and all our problems will disappear. I fell for every single advertisement going – the ones that told me their product was an indulgence but I deserved it and the ones that told me their product was revolutionary and would make me slim. I swallowed it all. Whoever snuck the 's' into 'fast food' was a sneaky little prick.

Why does losing weight have to be so feckin' hard? I mean, how many bleedin' scientists are there in the world these days? And not one of those nerds has come up with a magic pill that we can all take and then eat whatever the hell we like and stay slim?! I find that hard to believe. I used to be convinced that they had them in Area 51 and they just never told us about them. Bastards. The fat cats in the food industry want us to keep consuming so they get rich, but I guess the pharmaceutical industry must be more powerful because they want us to stay fat and unhealthy, so then we all get sick and have to spend a fortune on medication.

Back in my heavier days, if I had run for election to be president of the world, my main proposal would have been that they release the magic pills from Area 51 and charge us all a fortune for them so the pharmaceutical industry's hungry cash-flow would be satisfied, and the food industry would also be happy as we'd probably end up spending even more money feeding ourselves if we could eat whatever we liked with no fat consequences. I would have paid any amount of money for my monthly supply of magic pills, even if it meant I had to live in a cardboard box. At least then I could sit inside it, be slim and stuff my face with sugary donuts and double-cheese pizza with a gigantic smile on my face. Oh, if only it was that easy. I've done some serious research and it turns out there are no magic pills. The only thing that does it is hard work. Not the answer you want to hear, I know, but as they say hard work pays off. And when you sort out your head, cashing in is easier than you'd think.

The older and fatter I got, the more disillusioned I became with my looks. I've lived through the birth of the supermodel, the upheaval of the Wonderbra and the creation of Photoshop, where everyone is subjected to airbrushed skin, microscopic waistlines and legs so long the poor models would have toppled over immediately if they were that length in real life. And yet this is portrayed as the ideal, and we are led to believe that if we didn't look like this fantasy, then we are pretty much no better than a dog shit that has been baking in the summer sun. Pamela Anderson brought along her big fake tits in the 1990s and sprouted a sea of boners in the trousers of men around the world and us poor normal-titted chicks felt crap because we couldn't afford the boob jobs. What happened in the noughties? What were we supposed to ideally look like then? I can't even remember. I've lost track. Now we're in the decade of the big booty, where you have to look like you've stuffed two basketballs down the back of your jeans in order to be sexy and it doesn't matter what size your boobs are now because anything goes. And so the cycle of sexiness goes on. What'll be next? Will shoulder-pads come back? Or hairy bushes again, like in the 1970s? Or perhaps female bald heads will be all the rage just because some random fashion designer says 'They're so in for spring summer 2017 dahling!'? What a load of bollocks. It's taken me 36 years to realise that fashion is a load of shite. It's just a parade. I just want to be normal. I want to look like the best Jules I can and just be slim, healthy, fit and do a bit of decorating of myself with make-up and hair and not succumb to the latest cultural hype as to what's hot and what's not. Feck that.

Over the years, with my exterior deforming, inside my head was also morphing in the wrong direction. My mind and thoughts had turned from the blissful, carefree serenity of youth with no responsibilities, where my only agenda was fun, to a dark pit of despair where my thoughts were consumed by my appearance as I was failing miserably to succeed in doing anything about it. In this dark pit a weed grew, a big witch of a weed, the kind that would strangle a tree. This was the voice of my inner bad bitch. This voice would berate me day in and day out, telling me how fat, disgusting, ugly, cellulitey, flabby, vile and horribly gigantic I was. And it wasn't just when I was looking in the mirror, it was all the time. The more I tried to control the voice by going on diets to suppress it so it would have nothing to talk about, the worse it got. And that is because I am shite at diets. Absolutely shite. I have the willpower of a toddler in the sweets aisle. Did you know that diet stands for 'did I eat that?' I have tried so many and while I might miraculously lose ten pounds, as soon as I'd throw my bingo wings in the air to celebrate I'd lose my grip of the reins, my willpower would gallop off and I'd fall off the wagon, tumble down into a ditch, land on a sandwich, be seduced by the delicious bread and cheese and instantly make love to it. Then a few weeks would pass and I'd wipe the crumbs off my deluded face, get on the scales and see that I'd put back on the ten pounds I'd lost plus another five in interest.

This has been the story of my life for the past 15 years in fat jail. Normally a prison cell has concrete walls. Mine were covered in mirrors. Everywhere I turned, all I could see was my overweight body. There was no escape from the reflection as I desperately travelled through what felt like one of those warped hall of mirrors you'd find at a funfair. Yet there was no fun involved in my labyrinth of mirrors. All I could see was flab. And there was no exit sign or map either. I was lost and the slim me felt completely trapped in my fat body. I wanted my body to be a temple, but it was a bouncy castle.

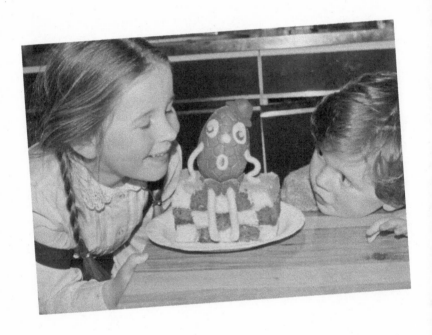

# 1

# Thick as Thieves

If I was to measure out every single alcoholic beverage I've drunk in my 21 years of boozing, I reckon I could fill an Olympic-size swimming pool to overflowing. It's a wonder I have any memory left after obliterating so many brain cells with all the vodka I've gleefully consumed over the years. My favourite drink is a lot. I can hardly remember what I did yesterday, let alone what happened in my early childhood.

Thankfully, my lovely mum documented my life in what we call my Baby Books. These are essentially diaries recording landmark moments in my life, funny things I said or did, stop-the-clock interviews, notes of achievements and, of course, the times when I was bold. I have eight Baby Books, spanning from birth to the age of 22. As my baby teeth fell out, they were carefully sellotaped into the book. When I swallowed some nuts and bolts as a toddler (as you do), they were fished out of the potty, rinsed, Dettol'd and taped in. Photos, letters, drawings, you name it, were all glued into the book. Mum was keeping Pritt Stick in business. These books are priceless to me and I'm very grateful to Mum for keeping a record of my life. She must have known that one day I was going to write this book and would need them as a trusty resource.

So let's do a full Craig David. Can I get a rewind? I was born on 9 August 1979, as Julie-Ann Coll, in Holles Street Hospital, Dublin, weighing a conventionally healthy eight pounds and one ounce. My parents, Jan and Mike, were both 26 years old. Mum was a film editor, and Dad ran his own printing business. I didn't get a middle name when I was christened because Julie-Ann was considered long enough, but my nickname, Jules, was adopted from an early age. We lived in Shankill in South County Dublin. The house was so small you'd put the key in the front door and smash the back window. It didn't matter though. Our little family was happy together and I was doted on. Thanks to Mum's Baby Books, I can prove this categorically.

Mum gave up work to look after me full-time and to say that she was a devoted mother is an understatement. I was stimulated with books and words and picture cards from an early age. I was on course to be the next Einstein, for sure.

*6 November 1980. Age: 15 months.*

At 15 months your vocabulary is now 115 words and each word you speak is very clear and distinct.

*17 January 1981. Age: 17 months.*

At the January sales in Switzers there were people everywhere. You were really annoyed at the big crowds. I looked down at the buggy and you were flailing your arms swotting people out of the way while shouting 'Christ! Christ!'

*22 March 1981. Age: 19 months.*

At 19 months you can read and say all the letters of the alphabet and you can read and count to ten. You speak in sentences of up to five words and include such words as deodorant, inverted and condensation. The progress in the past few months has been amazing.

I was breastfed for my first year and then all my food was homemade in true 1980s style: in the pressure cooker. This was all part of Mum's devotion to her children – she home-cooked and fed us as well as she could in the era of boil-in-the-bag curries and Findus Crispy Pancakes. So that's how I remember it – home-cooked food, largely healthy eating – which is why reading my Baby Books now, at the age of 36, I'm astonished to note how many references there are to food, weight and my undeniable obsession with sweets. For example, Mum writes that she had me on a diet when I was 18 months old because I was so chubby. I don't recall seeing any photos of me as a fat child. I was always slim and healthy-looking, so I guess that must have just been baby fat, which I eventually shed. Phew!

*3 December 1983. Age: 4.*

Jules: 'What does God do all day?'

What am I supposed to reply to that?!

Always an inquisitive child, I soaked up all the education Mum and Dad provided me with and I started primary school having just turned four and already able to read, write and count with ease. However, my teacher had to ask Mum to slow down on the extra-curricular teaching as I was ahead of the rest of my peers and was getting bored in class. Knowing me, I was probably sitting there filing my nails while staring out the window. I was nearly ready for my Junior Cert exams when I was only in Junior Infants.

*18 July 1984. Age: Nearly 5.*

Your class and Senior Infants went on a tour to Ashbourne to see a farm. It was your first tour and there was great excitement. Teacher gave everyone an orange juice drink, a Wagon Wheel and sweets. You said, 'I stood on a cow's poo and I ate so much I was as sick as a dog and Rachel O'Grady puked everywhere on the bus!'

*17 August 1984. Age: 5.*

'Mummy, I saw a bluebottle outside by the bins. He was a wild one!'

'How do you know he's wild?'

'Oh I could tell by his eyes!'

On our chunky 1980s stereo, Mum would record me and my brother, Barry, who is two years younger than me, on a cassette tape singing nursery rhymes and talking shite. We loved it and used to listen back to ourselves over and over again, thinking we were hilarious. One of the recordings has Barry aged just two, with his adorable lisp, strumming away on his toy guitar with plastic strings and singing 'Do They Know It's Christmas?' by Band Aid.

*12 October 1984. Age 5.*

This was probably the most moving tragedy I've ever come across. Millions of people in Africa starving to death because they haven't had rain for seven years and consequently can't grow their crops. The television coverage was so intense that there was hardly a dry eye in the country and this prompted a huge campaign to raise money for Ethiopia. This year we decided not to give Christmas presents and gave what we would have spent to Concern. You and Barry emptied your money boxes and that came to £12.50 and when you think of it 50p will feed one child for a week, so 25 children benefited from your little donation, Julie-Ann.

*30 December 1984. Age 5.*

Band Aid's 'Do They Know It's Christmas?' This was a record made by all of the most popular recording artists in England. It was a song written by Bob Geldof. The record, after only five weeks on the shop shelves, sold over 2.5 million copies and is the biggest selling single of all time. The proceeds of the song will go to help the starving people of Ethiopia. We bought 20 copies and you gave them as presents to all the family.

I blame Bob Geldof. A year after he encouraged us to 'feed the world', USA for Africa released their charity track 'We Are The World' – coincidence? It was all of this (as great as it was that they were raising money to help the people in Ethiopia) that led to every Irish mammy employing the phrase, 'Now you'd better finish everything on that plate! There's starving children in Africa who have nothing to eat for their dinner! So you'd better be grateful that you have food there in front of you! Do you hear me now? I want every scrap of that eaten so it's not wasted!' Every child in Ireland was burdened with the belief that it was a sin to leave food on your plate and even if you weren't hungry, or were already full, you'd better lick that plate clean or Mammy was going to phone up Bob Geldof and tell him that you were an ungrateful brat and she was going to swap you for an African kid who'd be only too happy to eat the bacon and cabbage she'd spent hours preparing. I now purposely always leave something on my plate to counteract that brainwashing. While casually wasting food is obviously not okay, when you're full, you're full. If you leave some mash and a Brussels sprout on your plate, that doesn't mean Bob Geldof is going to arrive at your front door with your grateful African replacement.

*24 May 1986. Age: 6.*

To Bob Geldof,

This is half of my Communion money. I made my Communion yesterday. I got an awful lot of money so I want to share it with the children in Africa.

From Julie-Ann Coll

*29 May 1985. Age: 5 and ¾.*

First Irish Dancing Feis

You got 2nd place and a certificate for the reel and jig. It was bedlam all round. When you were highly commended for the reel, you got a cert and you said 'I hate it!' You wanted a medal. Well, your dream came true when you got a trophy a little while later for the jig. Oh we were thrilled! Barry was bored stiff and moaned all the time 'I want more Bacon Bites!' It was an experience to see the Feis in action. Well done!

*June 1985. Age: 5*

Senior Infants School Report

Julie-Ann has worked steadily this year and has made very satisfactory progress. She is enthusiastic about her work and gives it her best effort. However, she finds failure difficult to accept and gets upset if she does not succeed. She is a very good mixer and is a popular child with the other children.

This report amazes me. Looking back on my life, I thought I just played and had the craic all through my childhood and teens and only really developed and fully became who I am when I reached adulthood. I thought I only refined my full personality then, but reading that I found 'failure difficult to accept' at the tender age of five years old really surprises me. I was obviously a determined little wagon even back then and if things didn't turn out the way I wanted them to, I'd get upset. Thirty years on and nothing's changed.

*18 June 1985. Age: 5.*

'What religion are you, Julie-Ann?'

'Book 4.'

*15 September 1985. Age: 6.*

When we were doing your homework on religion, we read a story about a boy who was watching television and his mother asked him to go to the shops for milk. The question at the end was 'What would you do?' You thought for a while and then said 'Well, I'd watch half the programme, go for the milk and have the rest of the programme recording on the video while I'm away and then I'd watch it when I get back.' I was speechless!

*22 August 1987. Age: Nearly 8.*

We went to the zoo. You moaned all the time. 'I'm too hot … I'm thirsty … I'm hungry.' You wouldn't take your sweatshirt off because everyone would see your vest. You were boiling and in the end I had to pull the sweatshirt off you. This was your third visit to the zoo and Barry's first. Mike made us laugh when he shouted 'Look, there's Nana!' – it was a rhinoceros!

I vividly remember this. I even remember the exact Snoopy sweatshirt I was wearing. It was one of those oversized thick ones that was like wearing a duvet. And it was reversible, so when one side got covered in chocolate dribbles and grass stains you could turn it inside out and have a clean, fresh sweatshirt in seconds. What an ingenious idea that saves the clothes washing by 50%. Everything in life should be reversible. As the sweatshirt was so warm, I only wore a vest underneath it and on that unexpectedly baking hot day at Dublin Zoo, I was sweating like a cat trying to bury a shite on a marble floor. There was no way I was talking it off though, in case anyone saw me in just my vest. I distinctly remember the feelings of panic and desperation at being so sweatily hot, but stubbornly insisting that it stayed on … until Mum pulled it off me to shut me up from moaning. She was dead right too. I am shocked that at such a young age I was so self-conscious. I didn't think that developed until I was in my teens, but it just shows you how early our self-perception develops.

Life was all sunshine and lollipops throughout my early childhood. As I got a bit older I seem to have envisioned some big plans for my future love life in millennium times …

*10 August 1989. Age: 10.*

Predictions for the year 2000: 'By then I'll be 21 and I will be in college if I get in. I will get married when I'm 25. I will marry Packie Bonner. We will have two kids.'

Fears: 'I hate spiders and burglars.'

Friendship: 'My best friend is Andrea. She is very funny and mad.'

Life: 'I love life, it's great!'

Love: 'I love hot dogs, Zig & Zag, Judy Blume, Fido Dido, Converse, Care Bears, Coke, Garfield and McDonald's.'

I obviously have always had great taste in men because Packie Bonner is still a ride!

*15 April 1990. Age: 10.*

Lent is over and I'm so proud of you and Barry. You didn't eat any cakes, sweets, biscuits or crisps and your Lenten record remains unbroken. You lost weight as a by-product and you look very well. An inch taller than me and I might add I don't like that!

The guilt I feel reading this is immeasurable. Not the Catholic guilt, I have long since distanced myself from the Church. It's been so long since I went to Mass that if I heard a priest say 'Body of Christ', I'd be like, 'Ah thanks Father, I've been working out'. I always found Mass insanely boring, especially as a kid. All those stupid step aerobics of kneeling and standing while rattling off prayers and hymns, half of which I didn't know the words to. So I'd just make up my own words, to make it more entertaining as I sang along: 'Joy to the world, the Devil's dead! Let's all clap hands and sing! He set himself on fire, and now Jesus is King! And now we all get toys! And now we all get toys! And now, and now, we get free toys!'

No, the guilt I feel is for all the Lents when I didn't actually give up sweets. In fact, Rick Astley gave up more than me. Naturally I claimed to be a Samaritan sacrificer and did some Oscar-winning acting at home, assuring Mum and Dad that I was sugar-free and that not one E-number had passed my lips for 40 days and 40 nights, making me big-time deserving of my Easter eggs as soon as Jesus rocked out of his tomb. The thing was though, while I wasn't having any sweets in front of the parentals, I was a right little greedy Zacchaeus scoffing the whole corner shop at five minutes to nine, Monday to Friday, before school started. I felt so guilty, even back then, but the temptation of Stinger bars, Black Jacks and Fizzy Cola lollies was too much for me and I was willing to risk the wrath of God and the fires of hell for my morning sugar rush.

I remember buying whatever sweets I could afford with the 30p in copper coins I'd managed to rustle together from down the side of the sofa or inside the Hoover bag. As I stood at the counter, watching the lady count out the penny sweets and hoping she'd throw in some extra ones for free if I smiled nicely, all the while I'd be anticipating a firm hand on my shoulder, then turning around to see Mum or Dad standing there with a look of disappointment on their face. Of course, I had my line prepped. I was going to innocently say, 'Oh, I forgot it's Lent!' I had actually practised the look of angelic innocence in the mirror at home.

Luckily, I never got caught, but I do remember one year breaking Lent so many times that I thought God had decided to get revenge on me. I convinced Dad to let me get an After Eight Easter egg. I wanted it because it came with a box of After Eights. An entire box just for me! Come chocolate day, I ripped open the packaging and inhaled the minty aroma. The egg itself was covered in shiny gold foil. I tore it off with vigour, and then my face dropped. It was dark chocolate. I hated dark chocolate by itself – with a minty fondant in a delicate After Eight, yum, lovely, but an oval of nothing else? Yuck. I was devastated. The box of After Eights wasn't any consolation. I had spent over six weeks dreaming of devouring this egg, all the time stupidly thinking it'd be milk chocolate, not the bitter dark stuff. And that's when I knew God was punishing me for being such a bitterly disappointing Catholic. Ah well, I'd try again next year. Here, by the way, did Saint Paul ever get a letter back from the Corinthians in the end?

My favourite books as a child were *The Emperor's New Clothes*, because there was a picture in it of the emperor in the nip and I thought this was just hilarious, and *The Magic Cooking Pot*, where the old lady made porridge in a pot that magically multiplied, so much so that the porridge overflowed through the village streets. I used to imagine myself opening my front door at home and seeing a creamy ocean of oats and gloriously diving into it with my mouth wide open. Bliss! I read all of the Roald Dahl books as I loved how dark and twisted he was, especially in *The Witches* and *The Twits*. I had a cassette tape of his *Revolting Rhymes*, which were gruesome versions of fairy tales where the alternative happy endings included Little Red Riding Hood shooting the wolf and thus bagging herself a wolfskin coat. (What a legend!) But no book made me eagerly turn more pages than *Charlie and the Chocolate Factory*. If I'd gotten a chance to dive into it, I would have been in that chocolate river like a world champion synchronised swimmer bringing home the gold medal for Ireland.

In fact, I had a real-life Willy Wonka moment in 1989 at our annual family treasure hunt. That year, the barbecue took place in glorious summer sunshine and my uncle, who worked for Cadbury's, was in charge of the prizes. Each family received a three foot by two foot purple branded box filled with chocolate bars and sweets. There must have been 500 Cadbury's products in each box. There was a riot in the garden as they were dished out. Some of the families had four or five kids, so they were all scrapping amongst themselves, stashing sweets in every available pocket and orifice before our parents, who were tipsy on the vino, could tell us to calm down and not eat everything at once. Luckily, in my family there was just me and Barry to lay dibs on our box. '250 bars each!' I calculated ecstatically.

I remember having a near-death-by-chocolate experience that day when I poured two packets of Creamy White Buttons into my mouth simultaneously and choked on them. I somehow managed to not turn blue by beating myself repeatedly on the chest, then swallowing them and shovelling in more. Myself and all my cousins were in chocolate paradise. Willy Wonka, eat your knob off!

Eventually, the box was taken off us and put in the boot of the car to be rationed out over the coming year. It lasted a mere couple of months. The coveted box was kept at home in the utility room. I had Barry well trained as my accomplice. He would keep sketch as I rifled through the Cadbury's goodies, grabbing as much as I could fit into my pockets, and then we'd run off up the garden and hide in the greenhouse and stuff our faces while laughing our furtive heads off.

We did a lot of sneaky sweet stealing over the years. We were like chocolate-thieving ninjas. I found the best way to get me to stop biting my nails was to tell me that Christmas was approaching. Then I would be well equipped to peel the sellotape off the lid of the tin of Cadbury's Roses that 'wasn't to be opened until Christmas week', take a handful and expertly replace the sellotape so it looked untouched. By the time Christmas rolled around, there'd only be half a tin of sweets left and Mum would be saying, 'They're putting less and less in these tins every year,' as Barry and I looked slyly at each other with Machiavellian grins. Our crafty ritual was disrupted one year when the tape on the tin was changed and it came branded with the Cadbury's logo. Our clear sellotape wasn't going to cut it as a replacement, so we had to improvise a new strategy. After much deliberation and endless strategy meetings in our treehouse, we decided it was best to very delicately peel off the tape halfway around – this had to be done with surgical precision, just enough to lift the lid a fraction, shake out some sweets, close the lid and then gently press the tape back into place. I still recall the adrenaline rush I would experience while doing this, praying it wouldn't tear.

My unrivalled abilities to defeat sellotape packaging often came in handy through the years. Dad did printing work for HB Ice Cream and he came home one day with a big box filled with tubs of ice-cream

Flabyrinth

and Magnums. This was 'not to be touched' as it was 'to last the whole summer' and was placed at the bottom of the deep-freezer. Again, Barry and I employed the sellotape trick, cleverly opening the bottom of the box so there'd be no evidence of our larceny. We had ice-creams on tap – fleecing them out and happily giving ourselves brain freeze whenever we saw a window of opportunity when no one was looking. Of course, one sunny day Dad went to take the box out of the freezer to give us a treat, and it was as light as a feather. Interrogation ensued, and we got into big trouble once we'd confessed to our almost-perfect crime.

My dad has a remarkable ability to delay gratification. This is evidently a legacy I didn't manage to absorb from the gene pool. On Sundays, the only day of the week we'd have a dessert, Mum would serve up either stewed apple and custard or a bowl of ice-cream with tinned fruit cocktail and if she was going all out it was Angel Delight with sliced banana – the height of 1980s-ness. Barry and I would have ours inhaled so quickly it barely brushed past our tastebuds, whereas Dad would leave his to sit in the bowl, sometimes for hours on end. After dinner, we'd all be doing the dishes together while dancing around the kitchen listening to Dire Straits or David Bowie songs and I'd be eyeballing his bowl of dessert safely resting on the countertop melting away. I could never comprehend how he had the ability to restrain himself from immediately devouring it when it landed on the table with the rest of ours. Actually, it's a wonder I managed to withhold myself from polishing off his Vienetta and telling him the dog ate it while he was drying the dishes! Dad had mastered the art of restraint. I was as instant as Smash.

Club Milk bars were our favourite thing to thieve. They'd come in a family pack of 15. We'd nick them three or four at a time. They were kept up in a high press in the kitchen. So one of us would keep sketch while the other hopped up on the kitchen worktop, delicately balancing on one foot like a well-trained ballerina, stretching out the other foot to rest it on the handle of the oven door. Then whip open the press, grab, jump down and go! We had it down to a fine art. When the Club Milks ran out, it was on to the dangerous territory of pilfering the KitKats. If stealing a Club Milk was a venial sin, then stealing a KitKat was a mortal one. Compared to the Club Milks they were easily accessible, sitting in the fridge door, but they were Mum and Dad's KitKats for their coffee breaks. There were strict rules around them and only when we got so desperate that we felt our sugar levels dropping into near-ketosis did we go for these and pray we wouldn't get caught, or we would have been killed. While watching TV in the living room, we'd unwrap our haul of contraband and casually shove the wrappers down into the crack in the side of the sofa as we munched away, delicately nibbling the chocolate from around the edge of the Club Milk, chipping away at it until just the interior biscuit was revealed and then that was duly dissected. Eventually, the wrappers would build up to such an immense collection that when you sat down on the sofa there would be a loud, very audible rustle of tinfoil and paper crinkling, at which point Mum or Dad would pull up the cushion, revealing the countless empty packets of irrefutable evidence and then yell, 'Julie-Ann! Barry! Get in here now!' As soon as we heard that, we would peg it out the back door as fast as our sugar-fuelled legs could carry us.

I know most kids idolise sweets, but I do wonder if I was even more obsessed than your average sweet-toothed child. I vividly recall Santa bringing me a toy sweet shop for Christmas when I was four. The first thing I did was rip the lid off the tub of hundreds and thousands and knock them back into my mouth. I don't understand it though, because it's not like sweets were alien to me. We were allowed to have sweets growing up. We had a Club Milk bar daily in our lunch-boxes. We got 50p after Mass on a Sunday to spend in the shop on whatever we liked. Mum and Dad were always generous with the 'Okay then, you can have a KitKat because you did all your homework in silence.' We weren't deprived. Yet I was bewitched by sweets to the degree that I was always wondering where my next source of chocolate or crisps was coming from. My nightly prayers included a request to Holy God that there would be no wafer in my KitKat so I could send it back to Nestlé with a well-worded complaint letter. I was specific about the KitKat because I knew Nestlé didn't just send you a measly two-stick replacement KitKat back in the post. Oh no, rumour had it that they compensated you with a whole packet of KitKats, sometimes two. And if they came in an envelope addressed to me, then I was sorted. I regularly reminded Mum and Dad that it was 'a federal offence to open someone else's mail', a handy fact I'd picked up from an American TV show.

*6 January 1989. Age: 9 and ¼.*

Dear Tayto,

I am complaining about my Monster Munch. They were stale. I kept them in a dry place in the six-pack bag. I opened a packet one morning and they tasted stale. It said on the packet best before 17th of February!

Very Annoyed,

Julie-Ann Coll

*29 January 1990. Age: 10 and ½.*

Dear Oatfield,

I purchased a packet of your Eskimo Mints in Quinnsworth in Stillorgan. When I opened the sweets, they were all crushed and in bits. I was very disappointed! Please find the packet enclosed as I would like a replacement. Thank you.

Very Upset,

Julie-Ann Coll

Barry and I would get up very early on Saturday mornings, go into the living room and make a fort out of the sofa cushions, cover it with blankets and then go into the kitchen to pour ourselves two gigantic bowls of cereal. I always chose the biggest breakfast bowl and filled it with cornflakes and Alpen until it looked like a muesli mountain. I would then delicately stick my finger in the centre of my breakfast volcano to make a well and pour in the milk ever so slowly to prevent it gushing down the sides of the peak and overflowing off the edge of the bowl. Then I would carefully carry the bowl to the living room, leaving a trail of milk all along the way, and Barry and I would enter our sofa fort, batten down the hatches and watch cartoons for hours.

We got on great growing up as we were just as devilish as each other. Sometimes we would pretend we hated each other but we didn't really. We even had a secret handshake. Refusing to shake hands with each other at Mass for the 'Peace be with you' bit because we were like, 'Ugh. I am so not touching your smelly hand it's probably covered in poo and snots!', we would instead just briefly touch the tips of our little fingers together. We still do it to this day. It's funny how that little ritual grew over the years to represent even more sibling affection than any embrace. (I know he'll read that heartfelt statement and say to me, 'That line made puke in my own mouth!')

Barry and I were a force to be reckoned with. Our poor babysitter, Kate from up the road, wasn't paid enough to put up with us. Jacked up on E-numbers from Skittles, we once took her shoes, filled them with pebbles and threw them into a bush of six-foot-high nettles, just for the laugh. At least poor Kate only had to endure us once a month for a few hours. I don't know how Mum had the patience to put up with our cunning plans day in, day out. I think she just laughed her way through it as there was no point in trying to dampen our spirit or our fierce determination. Any resistance would have made us even more resolute.

*6 February 1990. Age: 10 and ½.*

You have a bad flu at the moment and are confined to bed. You asked me to get you a Pot Noodle and of course I wouldn't hear of buying such rubbish so you wrote this note to Barry and asked me to give it to him:

'Barry, Get me a Pot Noodle at the shops. Bolognese flavour. You can have the change and two of my throat lozenges. £1 is in the envelope. Jules'

When he read the note he asked me was I going to Quinnsworth. I said, 'Maybe', just to add a little drama to the plan. We went anyway and when we got there, Barry said he'd be back in a minute. When he returned, he had the 'thing' in a bag. Really made me laugh. You would eat nothing but rubbish if I let you. You had the Pot Noodle and then spent the following day on the toilet with chronic constipation and you vow you're never eating a Pot Noodle ever again. Just proves how really bad they are.

I wonder how, when we consumed as much sugar as we did as kids, our waistlines weren't the size of tractor tyres. I think there are probably three key reasons for this: one, we ate a lot less processed foods than we do these days; two, in the 1980s the average daily sugar intake was eight teaspoons per day, which has now, in 2016, tripled to a whopping 24 teaspoons, four times the daily allowance recommended by the World Health Organization; and three, we ran around all day long. We moved to Carrickmines in County Dublin when I was six, to a house on an acre of land, so our new back garden was huge. We would bolt out the back door after breakfast and play with our best friends up the road, a family named the Berrys, for the entire day, only coming back in when we heard 'Lunch!' or 'Dinner!' hollered by Mum. We'd play Tip the Can and Army and Chasing and only a torrential thunderstorm with a threat of lightning electrocution would force us back inside the gaff.

The Berrys always had lovely things in their fridge and their mum, the coincidentally named Mary Berry, made the best chocolate profiteroles on the planet. They even had a SodaStream. I was so jealous. On rainy days when we weren't playing basketball outside, Mags, who was my bestie Berry friend, and I would spend hours in the kitchen pretending we had our own cooking show on TV. Our eye-line was to the microwave across the room, which was the 'camera', and we'd put on posh voices and guide the imaginary viewers through the recipe. Most of the time it was milkshakes or butterfly buns that we made and then of course we'd scoff them. We ate an entire apple tart between us one day and poor Mags was doubled over afterwards and had to lie down. I was grand and ready for seconds.

It's funny, the difference with kids today. We have a childhood obesity crisis now, and you'd have to wonder is it because kids don't run around as much as we used to? Is it because they're all glued to electronic devices while sitting on the sofa? We didn't have mobile phones or tablets back in the day. We could leave the house and be gone for hours, playing in the forest at the back of our garden, and Mum and Dad would never worry about where we were. Nowadays, kids have to text their parents every 15 minutes to let them know that they haven't been abducted by a psycho child snatcher. It's sad really, when you think about it.

Speaking of sad, would you think I was pathetic if I told you that I still sleep with my security blanket? Well, I'm going to admit to it because I love him. His name is Fuddy and he brings me immense comfort. I just love the feel of him. Sadly, he isn't my original Fuddy. My first Fuddy was the blanket I was wrapped in as a baby. He was pink, white, yellow and blue and made from soft wool. I would run his tassels through my fingers for hours on end. Over the years, he became shabby and Mum would have to sew him back together every so often. I would cry every time he went into the washing machine because I thought he'd drown. When I was 18, I went on a piss-up holiday to the Canaries with the girls to celebrate finishing school. Of course Fuddy came along too. We had to change apartments after being threatened by some looper man for reneging on buying tickets for a club night we decided we didn't want to go to. Crazy man came knocking at our apartment door shouting his head off. We were so terrified we changed rooms. In the scramble to gather our stuff, I forgot to bring Fuddy, who was tucked safely under my pillow. The next day, when I realised I'd forgotten him, I freaked and I desperately asked at reception if I could return to our room to get him. When I did he was gone. I was so upset. Mum got me a new Fuddy when I came home and reluctantly over time I fell in love with him just as much. Whenever Barry wants to piss me off, he says, 'Fuddy is being used as a cleaning rag in the Canaries! They probably use him to mop up shite in the jacks!' and nothing can cut me to the core more than the vision of that. Poor Fuddy. I hope he's okay wherever he ended up. And Barry, you're a bollocks!

I'd love to go back to being a kid again. Life was so carefree. No bills or responsibilities, the only thing I had to endure was school. I liked primary school, and loved meeting my friends by the bin to pretend we were sharpening our pencils so we could have a chat. I especially loved getting the job to go outside and bang the blackboard duster, and play-time in the yard was brilliant, but I hated school work. I found it tedious. I only liked art time, when we got to crack open the paints, put on our Dad's old shirt backwards and go bananas. Luckily, one year I had a teacher who was really liberal. Her boyfriend would call into the classroom regularly to visit her, with his dog, which was exactly like the one in the Dulux paint ad, and we'd all put on our coats and go for a nature walk in the local park so they'd have an excuse to spend time together and she could have a fag. That year our unconventional teacher didn't stick to the curriculum and we pretty much had free rein to do what we wanted each day. The nerds got stuck into their *Figure It Out!* maths books while I spent months making loads of campaign posters for Mary Robinson, who was running in the presidential election, and I hung them up all over the school. Girl power and all that. I think this freedom with art time is where my true passion for expressing myself creatively was born.

I'd always get a Pavlovian thrill when the bell rang signalling break-time and we all whipped out our lunch-boxes. I had the same thing nearly every day: a brown bread ham and cheese sandwich (sometimes it had tomato in it too, making it sumptuously soggy); a mandarin orange; a Club Milk bar; and a flask of Kia Ora orange squash. The odd time I'd get a banana, which would inevitably be made into a smoothie by my books at the bottom of my bag. I was always jealous of the girls who were allowed to have sandwiches filled with chocolate spread. Not a hope in hell Mum was smearing that on our sambos. On many occasions, to satisfy my tummy rumbles, I'd scoff all of my nosebag at little break and then hugely regret it come big break. So I'd have to scab my way around the class like Oliver Twist, to see if I could get my hands on any discarded sandwich crusts. Nearly once a week there was someone in the class who'd forget their lunch. It happened to me a couple of times and it was the best day ever as everyone would be asked to donate a bit of their lunch, so you ended up having a lovely little eclectic picnic.

Hands down though, the best day in school was cake sale day. This was amazing for two reasons. One, you got to make a cake to bring in for the sale, so I would always suggest to Mum that we should make buns instead – that way, she wouldn't notice if some went missing the night before, whereas a chunky slice taken out of a cake would have been more evident, but I wouldn't have put it past me. Once our buns were donated, we got to buy a cake at the sale. The best one we ever got was the Humpty Dumpty. It was almost too pretty to eat – almost. It consisted of a Battenberg cake cleverly acting as the checkered brick wall that Humpty was sitting on and his body was made from a chocolate Easter egg with iced legs, arms and face. Once Barry and I had posed for a commemorative photo with Humpty, all the King's horses and all the King's men couldn't put Humpty together again because Barry and I had decapitated him in a savage assassination with lashings of iced bloodshed until there was just some shrapnel of crumbs remaining. Smell ya later, Humpty Dumpty!

My best mate in school was Andrea; we'd been joined at the hip since Junior Infants. We referred to each other as Gertrude and Jacinta and just for the bants we would talk to each other in a strong inner-city Dublin accent. We shared a love of Care Bears, Bananarama and sweets. When Dad, whose company printed the tray-liners for McDonald's, was invited to the opening of a new McDonald's in Stillorgan Shopping Centre, there was only one choice as to who was going to be my plus one. Jacinta screamed, 'Are ya jokin' me, Gertie?!' with high excitement when I told her we were going to meet Ronald McDonald and we talked about nothing else in the run-up to it. At what looked like a swanky soirée to my youthful eyes, because all the adults were drinking wine in a fast-food restaurant, we ran up to the counter with the tenner Dad had given us to order our Happy Meals. Going to McDonald's was a rarity for us, so the thrill was unbelievable and our minds duly melted when we discovered that all the food was … FREE! Anything we wanted on the menu was on Ronald's tab. I turned to Andrea and told her, 'I'm gonna marry Ronald! He is the best!' and then rattled off my order to include, in addition to my hamburger Happy Meal, six chicken nuggets, a chocolate doughnut and not one but two ice-cream sundaes because I couldn't decide whether I'd prefer strawberry or caramel flavour. Needless to say, we couldn't polish off half of it and as soon as we got home, I puked like a garden sprinkler. Still though, best day ever. And a photo of myself and Ronald ended up in the newspaper the following day, surely a sign that he was my betrothed and we were going to live happily ever after?

While Barry was my accomplice at home for getting my pilfering paws on sweets, in school I formed an alliance with Andrea, who was my trusty accessory for toothsome missions. At after-school tennis practice, we used to purposely lob the tennis balls up over the fence so they disappeared into the field. Then we'd ask our instructor, Pam, for the keys to her car so we could get some more balls from her boot. Giggling hysterically like the brats we were, we'd open her car, rifle the ashtray for coins and sprint to the local shop to buy sweets. We'd be gone for ages and of course never come back with replacement tennis balls, just blue-stained lips from Mr Freeze ice-pops and sticky fingers from Dib Dabs. Thankfully, poor ol' Pam, who was trying to control a riot of other kids, never noticed. Or maybe she did, but was just thankful for a break from the two most disruptive tennis un-enthusiasts in her class.

By fourth class, when we were around the age of ten, the teachers started to notice changes in Andrea's behaviour and appearance. Every day she would ask me to bring in an extra flask of my Kia Ora squash, which I happily did because she was my bestest buddy. Until the size of the bottles started to increase to two litres. I thought it strange, but put it down to the fact that it must be thirsty work being my best friend as we talked a lot. When Andrea's weight dropped rapidly, she was taken to hospital. The doctor gave her a diagnosis of Type 1 diabetes. It turned out that extreme thirst was one of the tell-tale symptoms of the disease.

I had never even heard of diabetes and was very upset that my beloved friend was so unwell. I remember being shocked at seeing her frail state when I visited her in hospital. After reading up on it, Mum explained to me that Type 1 diabetes usually occurred in young people and the cause wasn't fully known, but that Andrea wouldn't be able to eat or drink sugar ever again. 'Oh dear. Well maybe it's not so bad. What's sugar in anyway?' I enquired innocently. Mum explained it was in anything sweet, like chocolate, cakes and our cherished Stinger bars. My jaw dropped. 'So Andrea's *never* going to be able to eat sweets *ever again*?!' I exclaimed in horror. Mum nodded. 'Sadly, yes. If she does, she'll be very sick. She'll have to prick her finger a few times a day to extract some blood and measure her glucose levels and she'll have to inject herself with insulin every day for the rest of her life.'

I was flabbergasted. I wondered if we were being punished for stealing from Pam, our tennis coach. And I also wondered if I too was going to get this dreaded diabetes. How did you catch it? Had someone sneezed on Andrea? Surely you don't get it from eating too many sweets?! In that case, I was nearly picking out songs for my own feckin' funeral. So as a mark of solidarity, and to cop myself on, I decided to address my sugar addiction by cutting down and I never ate any sweets when I was around Andrea.

Looking back, I think that addiction starts in the cradle. When we are babies, we are appeased with a breast or a bottle of milk or the aptly named soother (pacifier, if you're stateside) I had a soother until I was four years old. I called it my 'DoDo' and I vividly remember Mum telling me I was far too old for it and it had to go. She was absolutely right. I was flippin' four! Thank God I skipped playschool or the other kids would have wedgied me on a daily basis because of it. On a frazzled whim, my DoDo was swiftly banished by Mum and thrown out the upstairs bedroom window into the back garden. As far as my four-year-old mind could comprehend, it had disappeared into the abyss and I was thrown into a state of trauma and cried until I was blue, like the colour blue, not sad blue, well actually that too. Oh you know what I mean!

Anyway, my point is that it's clear to see that from an early age we are all consoled and comforted with food or with some form of soother because our parents don't want to see us in any state of distress. It's just the way it's always been. It's not the babies' fault, they don't wail their heads off thinking, 'I just have a lot of feelings!' They're just pre-programmed to get boobs or cry tryin'. Snappers, as cute as they are with their chubby cheeks and shite-filled nappies, don't come with removable batteries or an off switch. What else is an exhausted parent to do? Remember when we cried as kids and our parents said, 'I'll give you something to cry about!'? We thought they were going to hit us, but instead they destroyed the housing market.

So from an early age, like most people, I delighted in food, just with me it was always a little too much. I had no idea when I was a kid, as I was always slim, but I was basically a ticking time-bomb that would detonate in a further 20 years. In the meantime, I was busy heading for adolescence and hang-ups and a million distractions and anxieties, but thanks to my now firmly established obsession with eating, I was also unknowingly striding straight into the Flabyrinth in search of a new DoDo.

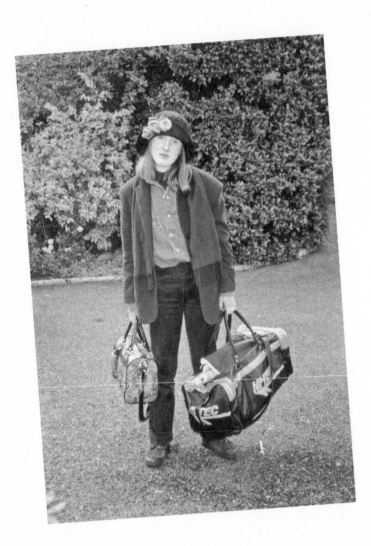

# 2

# Eejit Wonder

*4 February 1990. Age: 10 and ½.*

The school's retired principal told me today that I should explain the facts of life to you. I did!!! You weren't impressed one way or the other. All you said was 'That's weird' and 'Were you embarrassed telling me?' A few girls in your class have got their period and one girl got hers at eight and a half. Anyway with the help of a book called *Girl Talk*, it was quite easy.

*I*'ll tell you why it was quite easy, because I could have given 'the talk' myself. I was already fully swotted up on sex after learning all the ins and outs about it in the schoolyard. Andrea and I would giggle hysterically in the library as we'd flick through the pages of *My First Dictionary* to the 'S' section, then read the definition of 'sex'. It said 'male or female'. That was the extent of the description, but even at that we thought it was hilarious. We highlighted it with a luminous marker to help other kids searching for it in the future.

When I was in sixth class, it was a girl named Sylvia Hayden who was our encyclopaedia of sex. She knew it all and we were her keen students. God only knows what sort of misinformation she gave us and don't ask me where she got all her endless knowledge … actually, I remember! She had read Jilly Cooper's *Riders*. That was her bible. No doubt she'd fleeced it from her mother's bedside cabinet and she would relay all the facts of shagging to us at break-time as she sat there, like Jesus, and all of us her eager apostles with eyes and ears wide open. I can't remember her exact teachings, but I'd say it went something like this …

'Right. So you know a man's willy? You've all seen your brothers'—'

'—I've seen my dad's!'

'Ewwww!'

'Anyway, when a man sees a lady and he really likes her, his willy goes all tingly and you know the way it's normally floppy? Well, loads of blood, I think it's blood, or maybe it's wee, rushes into it and it fills up so much it goes hard and stiff and sticks up so it looks like a big aubergine sticking out of his body. When this happens, it's called an erection.'

'Go on.'

'So. When a lady fancies a man her fanny gets all wet—'

'—she pisses herself?'

'No-o! Stuff just comes out of her fanny to make it easy for it to slide in—'

'—for what to slide in?'

'The man's hard willy!'

'What?! The man puts his hard willy INTO her fanny?! That's disgusting!'

'It's not. It's very romantic actually. There's a special hole for it and everything.'

'There is no way I am letting a man stick his aubergine into my special hole! No way!'

'Well, I can't wait to get married and do it. It's meant to feel amazing and after he's stuck it in he slides it in and out for a few seconds and that makes the lady scream.'

'In pain?'

'No, in happiness. Then some stuff called sperm leaks out of his willy and goes inside her and that's what makes a baby.'

'That is sick.'

Thankfully, under the guidance of the *Girl Talk* book that Mum gave me, I learned how it all actually works. I read that book from cover to cover every night under my duvet with a little torch because I found the topic of body changes and sex absolutely fascinating.

*28 September 1991. Age: 12.*

You got your first bra which looks like a sawn-off vest, which we call a 'vra'.

I was absolutely dying to get a bra. All I had developed were two little budding breasts after praying nightly for them and rubbing holy water on my chest to try and speed up the process. At this age, I had just started secondary school. I had a slim body that had just started to develop womanly features. My armpits were bare and I had one pube, which I swiftly plucked out with a tweezers because I thought it was gross. My hips expanded overnight and tattooed my body with red stretch marks. I hated them and thought I looked like I was wearing a belt made of streaky bacon. I wanted that bra so bad, but I was too embarrassed to ask Mum if it was time for me to get one. Thankfully, the day arrived when she suggested it and I immediately played the too-cool-for-school act saying, 'God, Mum, I'm *so* not wearing one of those stupid things!', even though I was already practising for one by folding up my vest in half and modelling it in the mirror. 'I think it's time we got you one.' I rolled my eyes and grunted, 'God! Okay, fine then!' Off we went to Dunnes Stores, where Mum picked out a training bra for me: 'This is perfect, it's like half a vest. We'll call it your "vra".' Again I rolled my eyes and said, 'Whatever!' as I slinked behind a rail of clothes and grinned eagerly to myself while thinking, 'Yes! I've got a vra! I am so a woman now!'

Afterwards, we bumped into Andrea and her mum in the grocery section. While our mums chatted, I winked and nodded eagerly at Andrea and did some subtle charades pointing to my chest signalling to her that

I'd gotten it. She gave me the thumbs-up in delight as she'd already had one for months. We ran off and hid behind a clothes rack so I could show it to her.

*28 September 1991. Age: 12.*

What does a mother say when her 12-year-old daughter buys herself a baby's bottle on the same day she gets her first bra?

Don't ask me on this one. I haven't a rashers either. I must have gone into some sort of regressive state. I remember buying the baby's bottle with Andrea that same day, we bought one each and filled them with Diet Coke (no sugar for Andrea!). Now, why we did this I just do not know. My inner child was ready to grow up, but perhaps my inner baby wasn't ready to let go just yet? We must have looked like a right pair of oxymorons walking around the supermarket with those baby bottles and our vras at the age of 12!

With my vra finally manifested, my next nightly prayer was for the receivership of my period. 'Are you there, God? It's me, Jules.' I would check my pants every time I went to the bathroom to see if they looked like the Japanese flag yet. I'll always remember where I was the day that Aunt Flo visited for the first time and unpacked her red suitcases. I woke up feeling sick, but a different kind of sick. I wasn't sure what was wrong with me, but it was my first time experiencing cramps, I suppose. In school that day, we were doing fitness training for an upcoming 5K charity run. Normally I'd be bombing along, but I felt so queasy I had to go back inside. I thought I might be getting the runs, so I went to the bathroom and, lo and behold, Japan had finally invaded my knickers. I blessed myself and thanked God for answering my period prayers. Then I wondered what I was going to do about my bloody pants. I stuffed wads of toilet paper into the crotch and shuffled to the gym changing rooms, took 20p from my school bag and purchased a sanitary towel from the machine in the bathroom. Ensuring I had locked the door tightly, I unwrapped the pad and while humming Whitney Houston's 'I'm Every Woman', which was No. 1 at the time, I placed it in my pants. It felt like having a cotton canoe wedged between my legs and, because wings hadn't been invented yet, I was convinced it was going to slip out and land on the floor. I crushed my thighs tightly together and did the period penguin shuffle back to class, delighted with myself. At the end of each class that day, I stayed in my seat and was the last to leave the classroom, sweating with fear because I was sure I was leaking everywhere so I had to constantly twist my skirt around and check the back of it to see if there was a big red patch, but there wasn't. I would continue to do this for years every time I had my period in school.

There were so many worries that came with a period, like when you'd sneeze and then stay still while you figured out if you should casually run to the bathroom or if you were good to go. And of course, every woman knows the feeling of fear when you have to go digging for your tampon because you can't find the string and you panic that you've lost it forever and you'll have to go to A&E to get it removed! And the doctor will turn out to be an absolute ride and that'll make you even more mortified and you'd actually rather die of toxic shock syndrome than have him go hunting in your lady cave for your bloody tampon and have him pulling on the string and expecting the butler to walk in.

*22 March 1992. Age: 12.*

Characteristics: You love making lists. Organising picnics, labelling things, notes, e.g. 'Wake me up at 7 a.m. sharp! Have to wash my hair it's a major grease ball.' This is left on Mike's pillow regularly. You are becoming more inquisitive. Up to now you haven't been interested in anything adults say or do. School is 'thick' (your favourite word), almost everyone and everything to you is thick. You've started calling Barry a 'fart' even though you really care a great deal about him. You have your own taste in clothes, which I encourage. You like jeans, lumberjack shirts and brogue-type shoes. You have a few spots and your remedy for these is Dettol. You are a bit better at keeping your room tidy now that it has been done up. We have a good relationship and hug each other a lot but you won't let me go near you in public, although you'll hold Mike's hand. You haven't noticed boys yet, unlike some of your classmates who go to discos and even drink but they're very much in the minority. I would describe you as a very good-natured and well-balanced person. Because you are so tall people expect you to act older but you still have Fuddy! He's No. 1 and Quackers your duck teddy. You're doing well at school. You complain about the weight of your school bag. Two stone. Your pocket money is £2 a week and £1 for making the lunches. All in all you're a good kid. We love you and are very proud of you.

Once I had my period and my vra, I really thought I was winning at life. All I had to do now was turn 13 and then I'd be a fully-fledged teenager and that's when I'd be ready to take over the world. That's what I figured, anyway.

Much planning went into my 13th birthday. Mum asked me if I'd like a party. 'Parties are thick! They're for babies and babies are thick! I just want it to be me and Mags,' I told her. You see, I was still getting over the tragedy of my 11th birthday party. I had planned it to perfection. I got a bouncy castle and had seven of my best friends over. I had, of course, prepped all the sweets, crisps and drinks and had planned a meticulous schedule for bouncing time, casual chatting and refreshments. All was going great until I discovered that Anne-Louise, that stupid bitch, had removed the cling-film from one of the bowls on the table and started eating the Skips before the allotted time on my party itinerary. Well, I went mental and stormed off in a huff down the garden and sat with my back against a tree. Nobody came to get me for ages, I remember. Bastards. Eventually, Mags arrived and told me what I knew myself by now: that I was being silly. 'I hate Anne-Louise! I knew I shouldn't have invited her! She ruins everything! The thick pig!' Mags managed to convince me to come back and join the party as it was now officially 'refreshments time', so all the food was out on the table. Naturally, nothing was going to get me back inside quicker than knowing that. So I walked back in as if nothing had happened and hammered into the cocktail sausages while giving Anne-Louise the filthies. She was totally being 'skipped' on my next birthday invitation list. That'll learn her.

I went on about my 13th birthday for months in the run-up to it and somehow managed to convince Mum to grant all of my wishes as this was a landmark coming-of-age moment. For my birthday present I wanted the double cassette tape of *Now That's What I Call Music 22*, a pair of Levi jeans and a bodysuit. The bodysuit was a mistake though. The one I picked out had black-and-white stripes, I thought it was amazing, until I put it on and realised it didn't have fasteners at the crotch so every time I had to go to the bathroom, I would have to undress from head to toe. Pain in the hole! I may as well have just put on my swimming togs. Still though, I did look super-cool in my 30 x 32 high-waisted Levi's, stripey bodysuit, oversized grey zip-up hoody and black velvet hairband (in the 1990s this look was totes on fleek, I'll have you know!). My diva demands for the day itself included Mags and me being allowed to pitch the tent and camp in the back garden for the night and to have whatever I desired for dinner. So the menu was my death-row meal at the time: for starters, we had avocado with French dressing, which made me feel really fancy – avocados were expensive back then and not readily available in the shops like they are now; for main course, all I wanted was a Four Star Pizza.

We had never, ever had a takeaway delivered to the house before because Mum wouldn't hear of it. The closest we got was microwaved Marks & Spencer's chicken tikka masala while watching *Gladiators* and *Blind Date* on a Saturday night. So on this monumental day because, and only because, it was my 13th birthday, my wish was granted. When I phoned to order a large pepperoni pizza, I felt like I was a teenager in an American TV show. I could not have been cooler in that moment. But my hopes were crushed when, after giving my address, I was told they didn't deliver to our area as we were just outside the delivery boundary.

'Where does the boundary end?' I asked.

'Ballyogan Road.'

'But sure that's only one mile away!'

'I'm sorry but we don't deliver further than that.'

I did some huffing and puffing and told them we'd meet the delivery driver at the borderline in 40 minutes.

So off Mags and I set to burn off the calories of our impending cold pizza. I remember sitting on the wall, waiting, and jumping off as soon as we saw the branded moped arrive with our precious pizza. Hardly a home delivery service, but I was desperate and had a dream to fulfil and in all fairness we did live right on the edge of the sticks. We opened the box to take a peak and once the smell of the pepperoni and melted cheese caressed our nostrils we quickened our pace to get back home to devour it. The table was set for two. Not a chance Barry was getting a look in.

Candles were lit and Mum filmed it all on the home video camera (which I have watched back many times and cringed – this is how I know the details). Once the avocado was polished off, we divided the pizza between us while sipping on Aqua Libra, a fizzy fruit juice and the closest I was going to get to Champagne. For my birthday cake, I had insisted on constructing my own, which was a pyramid of sugar-dredged jam doughnuts. My favourite. I speedily blew out the candles and got stuck in. How, after the plethora of pizza, I had room to pack in more I don't know. We retired to the tent in the garden to listen to *Now 22* on my boombox and rub our overloaded bellies and no doubt talk about periods and the likes. Best birthday ever, until the torrential rain came down and we had to ditch the tent and go back inside. Sure my back was killing me anyway.

At 13, when my boobs were properly sprouting, I was obviously in full hormone production mode. Whenever anything saucy was on TV, I would cover Barry's eyes with my hands and jokingly say, 'Oh Barry! You can't see this, it's rude stuff!' and he would go mad trying to wrestle my hands away so he could gawp at whatever boldness was on screen. But I do remember watching the movie *Ryan's Daughter* on telly and in one scene where they were getting off with each other in the woods, it got really raunchy. The most porny thing I'd ever seen, anyway. In the heat of their passion yer man ripped open her blouse and exposed her boob. A nipple on the telly! Normally we'd laugh our heads off about it, but this time I didn't cover Barry's eyes. This time I felt different. I could feel something throbbing in my nether regions. I'd never felt that before. 'What does that mean?' I wondered. I hadn't discovered masturbation or anything like that at that stage. Maybe I was a late bloomer? But believe me, I made up for it.

Soon after that I started to become bewitched by boys. The only problem being that boys were alien to me. We lived on a remote road and I went to an all-girls' school. So being a prime candidate as one of those 'you always want what you can't have' type of people, I became obsessed. Barry went to Blackrock College and when we went to collect him from school, I'd be nearly licking the window trying to gawk at all the fellas. The second Barry brought home his school annual with all the class photos in it, I would hijack it and bring it into school so all the girls could drool over it. Most of the girls in school would hang around with bunches of boys they knew from their housing estate. Some girls had boyfriends. Sadly, in my gang of girls we were all in the same boy-less boat. I had never ever spoken to a boy my age and even though the thoughts of it terrified me, that's all I wanted to do.

I found this letter that I wrote, but never posted, to a problem page in a magazine.

Dear Kimberly,

We are a group of girls who go to an all-girls' school and we are in desperate need of men. We just don't understand it, we know hardly any guys and have nobody to hang around with. Let me just tell you that we are not really ugly and don't have non-existent personalities. Where can we meet guys? There are no cinemas, youth clubs, parks, shops or ideal locations around, believe me we've tried everywhere! Yet all the girls we know have groups of guys to hang around with. Please help us, we are in dire straits!

From women in need of men

P.S. Please don't go on about how important girl relationships are because we have ours perfected to a fine art! WE NEED MEN!

Oh. Jaysus. Imagine I went back and told my 13-year-old self that in 23 years' time I was still going to have the same shaggin' problem!

I became more self-aware at this age, because I wanted to attract boys, which meant I started to become more conscious about how I looked and began raiding Mum's make-up bag to try and make myself as ridey as possible. The first thing I experimented with was bronzer. It was called Egypt Wonder. Oh yeah, I want to look like Cleopatra, gimme some of that! It came in a little clay pot with a cork lid and inside was the magical bronze-coloured powder. I didn't know you were supposed to put it on with a brush, so I used the cork lid to rub it all over my cheeks and then looked in the mirror and saw a sunburnt lobster staring back at me. Mum came in and laughed her head off. You couldn't even tell how red with embarrassment I went because my cheeks were completely copper. I looked like Pikachu after a zumba class.

Mum, being the cool mum that she is, took me to the pharmacy the following day and I got my first foundation. It was a pot of Max Factor make-up crème. It was my new magical friend. Once I applied it, thankfully properly this time, I saw how it evened out my skin tone, made me look sallow and covered up the redness in my cheeks and the shadows under my eyes, and, most importantly, my horrible freckles were gone. I was enraptured. I soon realised that the more I applied, the more of a mask it created. Great. To complete the look I would smear kiwi lip balm from the Body Shop on my lips and clear, yes clear, mascara on my lashes and unplucked brows. That was all I knew then, I still had a lot to learn. I soon noticed everyone in school was wearing make-up. It was strictly against the rules, but we didn't care. I had to put my cream uniform shirt into the wash daily because it always had a terracotta collar by 4 p.m. I later learned why girls wore their school scarf all day long – it was like a handy sort of make-up-resistant neck brace.

At that stage school work still didn't interest me. I only liked Art and English – oh and Home Economics, but only when we were baking. My Home Ec teacher was a battle-axe. She wore more foundation than the entire lot of us put together. Her face looked like the surface and colour of that big Uluru rock in Australia. I bet she'd never even heard of cleanser and just trowelled on more every morning. I'll never forget the day the auld bitch had the audacity to ask me in class, 'Are you wearing make-up?' to which I replied, 'A little bit.' 'Miss Coll, make-up is strictly forbidden in this school! Go to the bathroom immediately and wash it off!' Mortified, I got up from my seat and went to the bathroom. I looked in the mirror. There was no way I was taking it all off. I'd become so accustomed to my fancy face that I didn't want anyone to remember what I looked like underneath it. So I decided to just rub a bit of it off with a tissue. I returned to class and sat back down. She came over to inspect me. 'I thought I told you to go and wash it off?' 'I did!' I replied. 'I meant wash it off with soap! Every bit of it! Get back down to the bathroom and this time scrub it all off properly!' The stupid cow.

I did as I was told. Nearly as bad as having to remove the make-up was using soap on my face. I was so into beauty products at this stage I was traumatised foaming up my face with dehydrating cheap soap. My face was red raw when I came back to class with my head down and the auld troglodyte Mrs Battle-Axe had a look of sheer smugness on her face. I wish I could go back now and have the balls to say to her, 'Fuck off, ya stupid auld bitch! I'm not taking it off! This make-up makes me look good and feel better about myself. At least I know how to apply it properly! Look at the state of your pebbledash face! You look like the surface of the feckin' moon with glasses and a wig on! Have you even heard of exfoliator?! Now take your panstick and shove it up your ratchety old hole! My foundation is staying on, okay?!' Oh, that would have felt amazing! Can't wait until they invent a time machine!

*19 February 1993. Age: 13 and ½.*

'Well Jules, what do you think of school?'

'I hate having to go to classes but I like lunch and break times.'

'Do you care about the way you look?'

'I hate my fringe. I hope it grows out. I hate my greasy hair and I hate having nothing to wear.'

'But you have loads of clothes!'

'I've got nothing! I've a couple of jumpers, a shirt, my waistcoat, my denim shirt. I've nothing!'

'What would you like?'

'I'd like a nice pair of platform shoes!'

'But they're only for scrubbers!'

'They're not! Everybody wears them!'

'What's wrong in your life?'

'My fringe. My legs. Janey mac, how could I forget Mr Kelly! He butchered me and gave me these braces! I feel like the Terminator. The fact that I have no money and any money I get has to be given away on stupid people's birthday presents!'

'What do you like?'

'Loads of things! McDonald's, Maltesers, clothes, Fuddy, watching the telly, playing basketball, toast and tea and chocolate.'

'What do you want to be when you're older?'

'I want to be ... I don't know. I'm going to marry someone rich and have loads of money.'

'Is money important to you?'

'Yes! Then I can buy loads of things I want.'

'What do you really want?'

'A swimming pool. A house in Beverly Hills. A pig and a sheep.'

'Who impresses you most?'

'Me!'

'What would you change if you could?'

'I'd abolish school!'

'What sort of man will you marry?'

'I'd like to marry a black man, he must be rich so he can fulfil all my needs. I'd like three children.'

'Thank you, Julie-Ann, for the interview.'

'I want to be paid for that now!'

As my make-up skills developed throughout the year and I learned to experiment more, thankfully with black mascara now, there was a landmark moment for my cosmetics training one day in French class. I even remember where in the room I was sitting when Chloé Browne walked in one morning and she had no make-up on, but she was tanned. I mean really tanned. 'Eh, sorry, Chloé, did you get a Concorde to Barbados and back overnight?! How the hell are you so brown?!' I couldn't understand it. 'It's fake tan,' she said smugly. 'Fake tan?' 'Yeah, it's my mom's. It's Vichy. It's like a cream and you just put it on your face at night and then wake up in the morning and you're tanned and it lasts for, like, a week.' 'Sorry, what?!' I exclaimed. 'It's like 15 pounds though. It's *trés* expensive.' 'It's cheaper than a flippin' holiday!' I told her. She warned me though: 'The only thing is that it smells a bit weird. Kind of like nachos mixed with treacle. So that's, like, a bit gross.' 'I wouldn't care if it smelled like rancid wolf shit! If I can wake up and look like I've been on holidays for six weeks while just lying in my bed, then I would endure any sort of toxic pong. Where can I buy it?' I desperately enquired. 'Oh in, like, any pharmacy.' Well, when Mum picked me up from school that day I told her we were going straight to Stillorgan Shopping Centre and I was getting an early 14th birthday present.

I had never known such a magical product existed. That evening, I squirted it out of the tube onto my fingertips. It was a white cream. I wasn't expecting that so I double-checked the label. Yep, I'd bought the right one so I trusted that if it worked for Chloé, it would work for me. I smeared it all over my face and neck. It stank. Chloé was right. Nachos covered in treacle. Cheesy nachos. I didn't care. I went to bed lying flat on my back like a corpse and hoping I wouldn't roll over in the middle of the night and wake up looking like Two Face from *Batman*.

I woke up the following morning forgetting I had the fake tan on and wondering what the awful whiff was. I figured I must have just released a lethal fart that had been trapped under the duvet. Bleary-eyed, I got out of the bed and went to brush my teeth. When I looked in the mirror, all I saw staring back at me was two white eyeballs and white teeth. I had transformed into Cleopatra overnight. Praise be to the Sun Gods! I jumped into the shower and reluctantly washed my face, thinking it was all going to disappear down the drain. When I looked in the mirror again, I was still brown. 'This is the best thing that's ever happened to me,' I thought. I strolled into school with a Rastafarian-style spring in my step and in the corridor I met 30 more Oompa Loompas, all just as ecstatic as me. Let's see Mrs Battle-Axe try and get us to wash this off our faces! Ha! Suck on that, biatch!

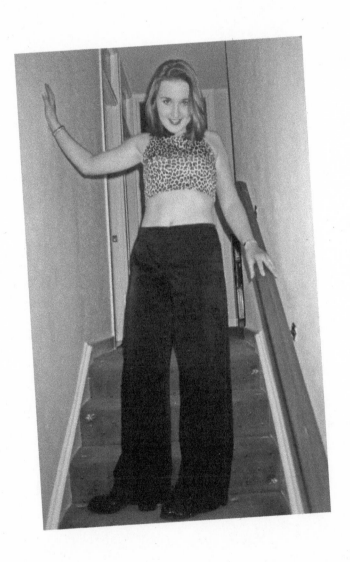

# 3

# Whore Moans

*14 September 1993. Age: 14.*

Your wedding prediction: Age approx. 24/25. Wearing an ivory dress with white Caterpillar boots with mint green or peach bridesmaids. On a tropical island paid for by your photography company. Bungee-jump off a bridge in your wedding dress. Reception at Tiffany's in New York. For starters: Salmon mousse. Main course: Macaroni and cheese sauce. Dessert: Christmas pudding with cream and custard. Drinks: Pepsi Max. Groom: Dark skinned or black. Mid-length hair. Curly. If a black man it must be in dreadlocks. Must be funny, loaded and play basketball.

y the age of 14, my desperation for a kiss from a boy had reached new heights. I spent an inordinate amount of time in school scrawling on my homework notebook about celebrities I was in love with and thus refining the definition of my dream man. I decided my hybrid He-Man should have the cuteness of Mark Owen from Take That, the coolness of Kurt Cobain, the looks of Robbie Williams, the attitude and poetic skills of Tony Mortimer from East 17, the dance skills of Howard from Take That, the funkiness of Jay Kay from Jamiroquai and that he should be a twin, like Bros, so I would have two of them to entertain me all day long. I drained numerous coloured pens doodling all over my books and folders in class. Then something happened, don't ask me what, ask that nut job Mother Nature, and the hormones in my body catapulted to new levels. I began fantasising about sex all the time. It was my favourite topic of conversation and the girls and I would eagerly discuss all things raunchy over sandwiches and Capri-Suns at break-time.

One day in secondary school, we got our 'birds and bees' chat. It was to be an update on the one we'd all received in primary school where they told us the basics. 'I could get up and do this talk myself,' I boasted. Fifty giddy girls were piled into a classroom where Barbara, the sex ed lady, showed us a really corny video explaining sexual intercourse. We were all in hysterics, sniggering away as it played. Afterwards, Barbara handed out pieces of paper and told us that if anyone had any questions that they were too embarrassed to ask, then they could write them down and she'd collect them in a box and answer them. Acting like I was the Fonz, I tore up my slip of paper as I didn't have anything to ask. I knew it all. Some of the questions were things like, 'Do you get pregnant every time you have sex?' or 'I'm 14 and I still haven't gotten my period yet. Is there something wrong with me?' I sat beside Sorcha rolling my eyes and mock yawning at the boredom of all of this. The next question was, 'What's a blowjob?' My ears perked up. Hang on a minute, I don't know the answer to this one. How come I haven't come across this? Barbara explained that a blowjob was a slang term for oral sex. For what? Oral sex? Again, I was baffled. She then went on to explain blowies in great detail. My mouth was hanging open. I thought it sounded horrific. I turned to Sorcha, 'Did you know about this?!' 'Ye-ah! Did you not?' she replied. 'No I bloody well didn't! A dick in your MOUTH?!' I was horrified.

That afternoon we were all as horny as bulls in a field of fresh goat weed. I couldn't get the vile image of a blowjob out of my head. I decided there was no way I was ever, ever doing it and instead I chose to stick to the romantic fantasy of sex that I had in my head. So much so, I decided to start writing about it. It started off innocently enough with short notes in my friends' homework notebooks, where I'd write out a little sexy scene for them about whoever they fancied at the time. The girls loved it and I loved writing it. So I decided I would expand my indulgence and express myself in the form of erotic novellas. Looking back on it now, it's gas, but at the time it was very serious business. I blame hormones for it all. The hormones made me do it and for a period of time I was so consumed by all things titillating that I appear to have lost my sanity, yet somehow managed to dodge being whisked away by the men in white coats.

As proof of my unhinged mental state, I am going to share with you an extract from *Steam*, my debut erotic musing. Other titles in this saucy collection include *Sweat*, *Moist* and *Saturated*. Luckily, I kept them for all these years. They are all hand-written and the book cover for *Steam* reads: 'Outside it's raining, but inside it's wet', which is in fact a line from the East 17 classic that gives the book its title. It also comes with a health warning stating: 'It's not advisable for people with heart conditions to read this.' The book itself is credited to Julie-Ann Coll U.S.M., which baffled me for a time until I remembered that U.S.M. stood for 'Ultimate Sex Machine'. So I obviously had quite the high opinion of myself and my sexual knowledge, even though I was a virgin. So finally, after 22 years, I'm going to give this raunchy tale the public unveiling it never had. We all love a bit of durt, don't we? A penny for your thoughts or a fiver if they're dirty and all that! But before you begin reading, I'd ask you to remember that I was a 14-year-old horny plonker when I wrote this and positively delusional with oestrogen. And given my quaint suburban upbringing, my experience of sex at this stage extended no further than seeing that nipple in *Ryan's Daughter*.

I imagine him naked in the shower. The warm, gentle droplets of water trickling down his body as the clouds of steam surround him. His hair all wet and stringy and hanging around his face. His eyes caress me as I look into his and melt into a mellow pool of rippling waves of lust in a sea of love. And then his hand reaches out and gently caresses my face and then runs slowly down the side of my arm. He takes hold of my hands and pulls me towards him to join him in the shower. He kisses my neck and then my forehead and slowly moves downwards to my lips as rivulets of water run between my heaving breasts. After ten minutes of energetic tonsil hockey, we step out of the shower. He wraps me in a warm, soft towel, previously washed in Comfort, and guides me towards the bedroom. Laying me down like an aeroplane on a runway, he glides swiftly over my body launching like a shuttle into a universe of ecstasy as our minds and bodies fuse in an aura of passion. His erection creeps up like a cat waiting to pounce on its prey. Gripping tightly our bodies pulsate to the rhythm of the crickets outside the window. [*To the rhythm of the crickets? Which means he must have been rogering me like some sort of gigantic vibrator on maximum speed!*] The silk sheets ripple like waves in a thunderstorm. Our bodies being the cliffs that break their power. The flashes, the lights, everything seems to be moving slowly. Moving frame by frame, making this moment last forever. Swooping up and down the rhythm increasing. Higher and higher as our minds and bodies climb to their peak. The passion, the ecstasy, climbing and climbing. I moan softly with the agonising wonder of it all. I was the braille book and he was the hands and he used his hands to understand me better. He withdraws the physical fusion, but the mental fusion remains.

He guides me towards the bathroom again. The jacuzzi is waiting. [*How convenient.*] Our blood bubbles as much as the water. We enter the liquid of love. His arms wrap around me as he kisses my neck. His erection floats above the water like the mast of a sailing ship. [*Obviously I had just learned about similes in English class and I couldn't get enough of them.*] Sailing in our sea of love. He kisses me gently. Slowly our mouths lock and our tongues search endlessly throughout each other's mouths entangling into a knot that any Boy Scout would be proud of. [*What the?!*] Again he enters me like a bullet launching from a shotgun barrel. [*I think this is like the third time we've shagged in a short space of time. So he is obviously super-human or I'm just immune to chafing.*] He kisses and nibbles my ear. Our bodies press firmly together. Gripping each other firmly, we can't control our screams and pants of ecstasy. He kisses my shoulders as I lick his chest. I can feel our hearts beating in harmony, faster than the pitter-patter of the water of the jets ricocheting against us. Our bodies fit together like a jigsaw, with no pieces missing. Our love is like sailboat, sailing through a sea of passion and through troubled waters our love feels no pain. We stumble out of the jacuzzi still clinging on to one another, not daring to separate. [*That must have been some manoeuvre!*] He grabs a towel and wraps it around us.

[*So at this point we pause our sexual Olympics to watch a soccer match where, in this alternative reality, Manchester United are beating Barcelona 27–nil and Eric Cantona has scored every single goal. Then we switch over to watch the golf and apparently 're-enact every hole in one'. Don't ask me. I was obviously demented. We then go on to have Olympic-level gymnastic sex another six times in various locations. Before ...]*

Rolling around the bed my body feels out of control. We slide off the bed on to the floor. He swiftly lifts me up and guides me towards the patio doors. He opens them revealing the moonlit beach outside [*Convenient*]. He stands behind me and wraps his arms around my waist and nestles his head on my shoulder. Our bodily oils glisten in the moonlight. We hold hands and walk down over the cool sand. He bends down and picks up a stick by some rocks. Holding it firmly in our hands together we write 'Troy loves Jules forever'. We look into each other's eyes passionately and at the same time say 'I love you'. We smile. [*That is simply vomit-inducing.*] As I look into his eyes, his expression changes. I know what's coming next. [*Yep, you guessed it! More shagging because this guy must have taken about ten Viagras.*] I turn to run as he tries to grab my arm. It's difficult to run in the sand, but I slow down, because I want him to catch me. He grabs me and lifts me up in his arms. He starts running towards the sea. Laughing and screaming, I try to break away but I love the feeling of his arms around me. He runs towards the water and when the water is around his thighs he lifts me higher and higher and then drops me into the salty sea. The water rushes over my face as I plunge under. [*Absolutely no consideration for my hair and make-up. The prick.*] He drags me back up towards the surface. We both laugh. [*Oh yeah, because nearly drowning me is absolutely hilarious!*] I place my hands on his shoulders and then suddenly jerk him backwards into the water. [*No, surprisingly not jerk him off, just jerk him back into the water.*] He falls under. I can't see him for a second. Then I feel his hands around my ankles. I think he's going to pull me under but then his head emerges from the water and he starts kissing my thighs.

We walk towards the beach but as soon as we reach the sand we lay down and as he runs his hands all over my body 'I love you. I love you' he keeps repeating over and over. As we make love slowly and romantically this time. [*Then all the previous shags were, I assume, buckin' bronco style?*] I know I love him. I cry out as wave after wave of intense pure ecstasy washes though my body. He clings to me. I rest my head against his chest. We are bathed in sweat and I can feel his heart throbbing, pounding, thundering behind his ribs.

[*I obviously consulted the thesaurus for that line and couldn't make up my mind on which word to choose so I just used them all. So at this point in the story, which remarkably actually has a plot, Troy the Trojan sex machine takes me to Paris in his helicopter. It only takes ten minutes to get there, apparently. In the restaurant at the top of the Eiffel Tower, he orders for us in French.*]

'Chez moi, Le Tour de France, bonjour, le frog's legs, le vin rosé, Irelande douze points, Channel Tunnel, Yves Saint Laurent, Cuisine de France.' I don't understand a word of it, but I'm impressed. [*He then proceeds to press a button and a red loveheart-shaped bed appears from the floor. This guy was smooth.*]

He takes me to the bed once more. He wraps his arms around me as we tumble on to the red sheets. Lying on top of me I love the feeling of the weight of his body pressing against me. Spreading my legs he grips the inside of my thigh. [*I think Troy must have gone to the cash 'n' carry to get the lube.*] I cling to the sheets as his rigid power tool drills through me. After some intense action, he withdraws and says in a whisper 'I've got a secret', giggling he tiptoes out of the room. [*Giggling and tiptoeing? Doesn't he sound like a right hunky Chippendale?*] He comes back moments later with a carton of Haagen-Dazs ice-cream. The bubbles on the carton remind me of the condensation on the window from the steam in this sweltering room. [*Bastard didn't even open a window. Lazy.*] He produces a spoon and feeds me some of the double chocolate chip ice-cream. It dribbles down my chest and he licks it off passionately. Then he delicately spreads the ice-cream from my neck down every crevice of my body to my toes. Feeling chilled, he begins to lick it off. His warm tongue removes [*didn't consult the thesaurus for that word obviously*] the ice-cream and leaves a shimmery glow on my body. [*A shimmery glow? I would have been a sticky mess! And we won't even mention the silk sheets. Who was going to clean those? Sure they'd be destroyed and if anyone had walked in it would look like a dirty protest.*] Then Troy looks into my eyes and says 'Will you marry me?' 'Yes! Yes! Yes!' I scream as he makes love to me. [*So I think that would be around ride number ten at this stage and remarkably there's still no mention of chafing or of Troy having to take a break to re-bone.*] After an hour, we were sitting up in bed together and I thought to myself 'Do I love him?' Questions ran racing through my mind. Who? What? When? Where? Why? Yes. No. No. Yes! I put the question to myself again and that's when I realised I didn't really love him, it was just our sex. A physical but not a mental relationship. [*That's probably because we never even had a conversation.*] No, I didn't love him. It couldn't go on. It had to end. It just had to end ... The End.

Holy sufferin' mother of perpetual succour. What sort of sex-crazed horny lunatic was I?! And who was this fantasy Robocock Troy who seemed to have an endless boner? I hadn't a rashers about riding and I think that's pretty evident. But the girls in school lapped up my bestseller, and I can claim it was a bestseller as I would charge them £1 to read it. 'Have you finished the next paragraph yet?' they would eagerly enquire and I'd tell them, 'Be patient. I'm a sexual artiste. These things take time.' As soon as the next instalment was down on paper, they'd be snapping it out of my hands while raining down pound coins on my desk. I had found my calling. I wish I had pursued it further. I could have been Carrickmines's own answer to E.L. James. But my publishing career was hindered by the interruption of distraction with real-life boys and real-life sexual experiences.

*Summer of 1994. Age: 14/15.*

This year you have become very close to your
cousins Debbie and Renée. You all seem to
have a lot in common i.e. horses, music and
BOYS. You have been spending all summer
hanging out with Gordon and Daniel. Daniel
it seems fancied you and you were completely
taken aback – this was your first brush with
boys. You drew insulting caricatures of them
and stuck them up in the local shop window.
Daniel and Gordon went mad and phoned here
to threaten you, but you weren't too worried.
Mike and I thought it was all moving too fast
so we had a chat with you. You thought we
were 'so five minutes ago' and 'not living in
the now' and 'I have to learn by my mistakes.'
You've grown up so much this year and we
know this is the beginning of bigger things –
we just hope you don't get hurt by some little
jerk.

Oh, the summer of Daniel and Gordon. They lived
nearby and spent most of their day kicking a rugby
ball up in the air. In order to get their attention, we too
started kicking a rugby ball while shouting 'I can kick
it higher!' over the hedge that separated us. What boy
doesn't react to a good challenge, eh? The exchanges
eventually led to a meeting through a gap in the bush,

where flirting began. Daniel, the more outspoken of the two, was sallow and skinny with dark hair; silent Gordon had *Wayne's World*-style shoulder-length black hair and a beard. They were both a year older than me and I found neither of them attractive, but I didn't care. They were boys. Boys I could talk to. Our initial dalliance involved a lot of joshing and slagging, but it soon turned to attraction. I didn't fancy Daniel. He was such a nerd. Yet he made me laugh and he used to write me long, hilarious letters and I found myself thinking about him all the time and putting huge effort into my spectacular reply correspondence. 'Oh God, Jules, you totally fancy him don't you? No, I so totally do not!' I would tell my in-denial self.

Here's an excerpt from one of 16-year-old Daniel's letters to me to show you what sort of teenage male I was dealing with.

A salut to those by the name of Jules. My watch is presently showing 00:37 which means that I should be in bed. The last two days have been more action packed than an episode of *Neighbours* (a Grundig production). I am now banned from two houses which are less than a mile from each other. Wicked!!! I'm banned from Ann's because I made a wanking gesture at Renée and I'm banned from Sean's because I set off his house alarm and had the cops up there twice in half an hour. Well ya know what they say, 'When the shit goes down, you better be ready!' Twice I complained about my summer being sadly boring but now it's gone stupidly to the opposite. Dig this, in the space of four days I have: met the cops three times, drank 30 pints of Bud, got kicked out of two humble abodes, got sick seven times, wasted £120 on nothing, had no showers (still haven't) and had to change my sheets 17 times (it's not what you think). I forgot to tell you what happened on Sunday, so I'd better spray some more ink on the page. At one o'clock myself and Gordon went up to Sean's house with TWENTY BOTTLES OF BUDWEISER. He wouldn't let us drink it in house, so instead we brought it all up to a cool waterfall place beside his gaff and emptied our sense into 6.6 litres of glass bottles. About two hours after that we emptied our stomachs into the river. Super mega hurl! At about four o'clock, back at Sean's house, I ACCIDENTALLY set off his panic alarm. It was kudostic! It sort of looked like Lautrex disco when it was activated. Red, green and blue lights were flashing all over the house, the movement sensors were bleeping like hell. Lasers were scanning across the floor and six high powered sirens were blasting a very monotonous tone in my direction. Wicked! Then when we heard the cops coming Gordon and I jumped through the kitty flap and broke the world record for the one-mile sprint (vehicles included). Gordon couldn't quite break the sound barrier – he was laden down with empty Bud bottles. When we got back to Gordon's we spewed a few more times and then watched re-runs of *Baywatch*.

For the laugh, one day I decided to put felt-tip marker to paper and drew unflattering caricatures of Daniel and Gordon and convinced Billy the local newsagent owner to let me put them up in the window of the shop. We waited with bated breath for their reaction, and they of course went spare. The following day Daniel shouted over the hedge and called me 'Holster Hips'. This cut to the core. I figured I must have looked like I was smuggling two concrete blocks down the sides of my knickers. I was already conscious of my changing teenage body and my now fully developed womanly hips, which had recently shot out like boomerangs covered in even more shitty stretch marks. I was a slim size 10 with B-cup boobs, a small waist and curvy hips, a figure I now look back on and see that it was absolutely gorgeous. If only I could go back and tell myself that I should have been strutting around in a bikini even when it was snowing, but I was so self-conscious as I graduated from child to woman that I kept it all under the wraps of baggy clothes, which, luckily for vulnerable teenage me, were the height of fashion in the 1990s. I was well able to dish out the slaggings in my uncomplimentary caricatures, but I soon realised I couldn't take the cheap shots when they slapped back in my face. I hated Daniel for that comment. Nobody had ever criticised my body or appearance before and it made me even more self-conscious. Myself, Renée and Debbie decided to snub Daniel and Gordon from then on. Yet I was always thinking about him. He had completely seduced me. The absolute bastard.

Even though I'd gotten the rough end of the stick with Daniel and Gordon, it didn't put me off heading back down the gauntlet of boys for more. What can I say? I'm a sucker for punishment. The first disco I ever went to was in a rugby club and it was a major let-down. It was too packed and I got chewing gum in my hair so we had to leave early. During school term it was difficult to convince Mum to let me go to discos, so, conniving little fox that I was, I would write letters to Mum to persuade her to let me attend. Well, I gave her no other option but to say yes.

*3 March 1995. Age: 15.*

Dear Mum,

I decided to write you a little letter as a token towards our mother–daughter bonding relationship. I may as well get straight to the point, you see the thing is I was talking to Renée on Tuesday and apparently there is a big Lautrex disco on this Saturday. And I was doing a bit of calculating using my top quality skills in maths and the last time I was in Lautrex was January 21st which was six weeks ago and in that six weeks I have only been out once to Bective last weekend (and I'm really annoyed I cleaned the kitchen and wasted the credit on that kip!) So I really haven't been out a lot. Renée and Deb have talked to Ann who says it's okay and they were begging me to come 'cos Lautrex just isn't the same without me! Who's going to dance to the Man United song with Deb? And who's going to do the 'Lautrex Walk' with Ren? Sure if I was in on Saturday night I'd just watch *Gladiators* and *Blind Date* same as usual it's not like we do anything special! Quote from you this morning 'Thank God I don't get any hassle from you Jules!' I don't really ask for much. I'll help you do another blitz cleaning job on some other room in the house as payment for it if you want? Thanks for being a great Mum and always listening to my side of the argument. Kiss, kiss, kiss, hug, hug, hug!

Jules xoxo

Tick the box: Yes ☐ OK ☐ Certainly ☐
Definitely ☐ Alrighty Then ☐ Sure ☐
Of Course ☐ Go on then you deserve it my
'no hassle daughter' ☐ Most positively yes ☐

The local disco, Lautrex in Greystones, was the place to be that summer. I went with Renée and Debbie that night in all our 1990s Lycra and sequins finery, with glittery blue eyeshadow to match. My Auntie Ann dropped us off and when we pulled in to the car park, up to ninety with excitement, noises came from the rear of the SUV and out popped Daniel and Gordon, who had hitched a ride by hiding in the boot. They thought we'd be delighted to see them, but we just looked at them with disgust, rolled our eyes *à la* Cher in *Clueless* and teetered off into the club. I found myself making eyes with Daniel across the disco for the night. Eventually, he plucked up the courage to come over. As soon as I saw him approaching, I immediately flicked my hair, folded my arms and looked the other way.

'Jules. Why won't you talk to me? What have I done wrong?' he asked. 'Don't give me that! You know exactly what you did!' I exclaimed. Baffled, he replied, 'I actually don't. I have no clue! Can you please tell me?' I swished my hair around and said, 'Eh, hello? You called me Holster Hips, you absolute asshole!' 'I did?' he replied. 'Yes, you did and I'm so not speaking to you ever again because of it. Now can you stand out of the way please because you're blocking me from view of all the guys who want to ask me to dance' (that would be no one). 'Well, what about the caricature you did of me?! You drew me with mountains of dandruff on each shoulder and little men skiing down them!' 'That was for comedy value. It was a cartoon drawing, not a portrait,' I said with utmost defensive attitude. 'Look, Jules, I'm sorry for calling you Holster Hips. I don't even remember saying it. You have lovely hips. Will you forgive me?' he asked. I paused for a moment and then replied while not making eye contact, 'Yeah. Okay then.' I flicked my hair again and continued to look anywhere but in his eyes. 'And are you going to apologise for the caricature?' he enquired. I grunted and rolled my eyes, 'Yeah. Whatever. Okay, I'm sorry. Are you happy now, you total smeg head?!' 'Jules, will you dance with me?'

Nobody had ever asked me to dance at the three discos I'd attended. The slow set was on and before I knew it, he was holding my hand and walking me onto the dance floor. My expression must have answered yes. I'd say I looked like a lost sheep in sequins. The song was 'Move Closer' by Phyllis Nelson. Daniel rested his hands on my holster hips and I put my hands on his dandruffy shoulders and we slow-danced. We were like two Frankensteins in love. My mind was racing: 'Oh my God, I am touching a boy!

We are actually physically touching each other. This is amazing!'

Immediately after that, we were apparently boyfriend and girlfriend. I became really shy, awkward and introverted around him. My previous ability to be myself and make him laugh with my cut-throat slagging disappeared. I'm not sure why this happened. He remained the same as always around me. Maybe I thought it was too good to be true so I was trying to prevent myself from messing it up? The mad thing is, I still do the same thing with men I fancy to this day (I really need to heal that). Eventually we knew our relationship had to connect further than holding hands and slow-dancing and we both knew when it was going to happen. The following week he was my date for my uncle's 40th birthday party, which was being held in a function room of the Royal Marine Hotel in Dun Laoghaire. I deliberated for hours as to what I should wear and decided in the end to go for a white belly-top with a blue checkered maxi-dress over it, a black choker and desert boots. The epitome of 1990s style. I thought I looked just like Tia and Tamera. We snuck out of the party halfway through to go for a 'walk' down the pier.

Again, my usual boisterous self was suppressed by reticence. Thankfully, he took the lead and we stopped by the yachts and turned to face each other. Oh God, this is it. We are going to kiss. Finally, I'm going to lose my snogging virginity. Prepare the fireworks! I was shaking with nerves. He leaned forward and we pressed our lips together. 'I've done it! I've kissed a boy!' I wanted to pause and run off and tell all the girls in school immediately. The kiss continued and I couldn't wait for it to develop into a proper French kiss, which it punctually did, and I thought to myself, 'I bet I look just like the sexy people in Hollywood movies right now. This is gonna be epic!' As we opened our mouths and began tongue twisting, I waited for the magic feeling to happen. But it didn't. 'Is this it?!' I wondered. 'Seriously? This isn't very exciting at all. Why isn't my leg popping up? It doesn't taste like I'd imagined. All this time I've been anticipating this moment and it turns out just to be a sloppy tongue sandwich? Snogging is so over-rated. Ugh.' It went on for a few minutes and I broke away when it didn't improve. I couldn't foresee tonsil tennis becoming a new hobby of mine. What a disappointment. I broke it off with poor Daniel shortly after that. Bitterly underwhelmed by the experience of kissing, I wondered if sex was going to be just as crap.

After my summer of disenchantment I returned to school and told the girls about my snogscapade with Daniel and of course made it out like it was so lascivious and passionate that we had to resist breaking into one of the nearby yachts to make sweet love to each other. It was transition year and I had been really looking forward to it as it meant less curricular and more practical learning, like first aid skills and trips away, but more importantly we got to do the school musical, *West Side Story*, with local school CBC Monkstown. Boys. Yes! Maybe I could find a boy there to do lustful things with? Fantastic. I was going to nail that audition, get the main part and then all the guys would fall in love with me. Bingo! I knew I could sing. Mind you, I'd only ever sung for myself, but I was sure the echo in my shower was similar to that of a professional recording studio and I knew that if any hot-shot record producers had happened to be casually strolling past my bathroom, then surely I would have been signed up on the spot.

All jokes aside, I can actually sing. I'm no Adele now, but I could have got a lead part in the musical if I hadn't let the nerves get the better of me. I practised 'I Feel Pretty' until I had it nailed. I was gonna go in there and blow their faces off with my powerful voice, snatch the lead role and then all the boys would want a slice of my slice. I was confident on the day, but when I was called into the hall for my audition, adrenaline crystallised my blood and I froze. The guy began playing the piano. I opened my mouth and honestly a sparrow with laryngitis would have sung louder than me. It just wouldn't come out. I panicked and that made it worse. This is why I now have to eat the cushions watching auditionees on *The X Factor*. I was raging with myself afterwards. My big powerful voice had been muted by my stupid nerves. When the parts were announced I was cast as 'Hot Dog Girl', meaning I stood in the background pretending to be a 1950s hot dog vendor. Yay. Well that's gonna have the fellas jippin' their jocks for me, isn't it? Sigh.

I still had a great time doing the musical and a lot of flirting took place. It was a hormonal storm during rehearsals. After our three-night run, the highly anticipated end-of-show disco was going to take place in the school hall. Everyone was out to try and lob the gob. I decided that I was going to give spit-swapping a second chance, just to see if it was Daniel that had made it a disappointing experience. 'I don't care who asks me, I'm just saying yes,' I told Mags. Fortunately, Marcus, a hottie from fifth year, asked me to dance. He was a total ride. Oh yeah, break me off a piece of that. Our slow dance followed that typical teenage manoeuvre. His hands on my hips. My hands on his shoulders and as the song goes on, we inch forward until we're chest to chest and ear to ear. Then we go into reverse gear and our heads inch backwards until we're cheek to cheek, signalling that it's time for mouth to mouth. This time it was different. 'The boy's got skills,' I thought to myself. 'Now this type of tongue wrestling I like!' This kiss went on forever. At one point, we had backed into a radiator. A boiling hot radiator and it was burning the shit out of my back, but I somehow managed to endure it for the sake of not wanting this magical snoggery to end.

But our passion came to an abrupt halt when the music stopped and the main lights came on revealing all the boys' boners and all the girls' panda eyes. Marcus and I said goodbye and Mags came over to me. 'Jules, he was gorge–' she stopped. 'Jules, what's up with your top?' I looked at her quizzically. 'What?' I looked down at my grey t-shirt and didn't see anything strange initially, and then noticed that there was a two-inch wet semicircle around the neck of it. 'Oh my God, Mags! Get my coat! Please! Quick!' Mags darted off to find my jacket (I still remember it, bottle-green denim with a lambs-wool collar), to save me from the mortification of anyone noticing that Marcus and I had DROOLED so much during our two-hour snog, which, shockingly, gave neither of us lock-jaw, that it had dribbled all down my neck. Gross, I know! But only me it could happen to. Only flippin' me. Mags arrived back in seconds with my coat, which I quickly fastened up to the top button. 'Jules, you need to check your make-up in the mirror too,' Mags told me. 'What?!' I sprinted like Linford Christie on hot coals towards the bathroom and found my face in the mirror. I looked like I had Michael Jackson disease because Marcus had eaten off all my foundation around the bottom half of my face. Cheers, Marcus! Hungry, were you? Did your mother not feed you dinner before you came out, no? Thankfully, I had more slap in my bag and I managed to patch up my pash-rashed face. Phew. Still though, that night was a result as snogging was back in my good books. In fact, it was my new favourite thing.

With my new-found taste for kissing, it became my full-time hobby. So much so, I had to start keeping a record of all the boys I'd locked lips with in my Him Book. I would note their details and give them marks out of ten for looks and snogging skills. The numbers soon started clocking up.

Snog Number: 35

Name: Robbie —

School: Grosvenor Park

Hair: Black

Eyes: Brown

Place: Outside the Bull & Bear pub

Looks: 9/10

Snogability: 9/10

He was wearing: White tight top, black Adidas tracksuit bottoms

I was wearing: See-through leopard-print shirt, black Wonderbra, brown suede mini-skirt, brown knee-high boots

## 11 March 1996

I've seen him a few times in the Bull & Bear
and I said that he looks exactly like Peter
Andre. I was up at the DJ box chatting to
the DJ, Fred, when Robbie came over and
requested LL Cool J's new song. I noted that
and when he was gone, I said to Fred, 'He's
a fine thing'. Fred said he's a really nice guy
as well. Never in a million years did I think
I'd stand a chance with him. Anyway, a while
later he came over and stood beside me and
started looking through Fred's CDs. I was just
foaming at the mouth and he turns to me and
says 'Any requests?' I nearly passed out and
had a stroke and a heart attack simultaneously.
Then I remembered the LL Cool J request so
I suggested that. He asked my name and I got
talking to him. He's so sound. I told him he
looked like Peter Andre and he admitted he
was a major fan. So, I was talking to him for
ages, he can really hold a conversation. He
can't get tickets for the Peter Andre concert,
it's so weird he's really into Backstreet Boys
etc. I told him I was a DJ on Pulse FM and he
was well impressed. He asked how I got the
gig and I told him I just wrote to them and
sent them a tape of me doing my DJ voice and
they gave me my own breakfast show for the

summer. It actually sounded so cool. I wasn't going to tell him I have to get two buses there at seven o'clock in the morning and it actually broadcasts from a shed in a back garden. I made it sound like I was a total pro and he was loving me cos I'm as cool as a deep freezer.

He has his own car, a little banger Peugeot, which he thinks is absolutely gorgeous, but hey it goes! He brought me outside to see it, he has a sticker on the back that says 'Damn I'm Good' which just about sums him up! He knows he's a babe but I was well able to handle him. I gave as good as I got on the scale of who's the coolest. We were standing beside Mags's car and I was saying 'Oh I'm so cold' (hint hint) and he put his arms around me and kissed me. I cannot believe I was with a Peter Andre lookalike. I was only with him for about five minutes because Mags and Sorcha came out. He asked what I was doing tomorrow. I told him nothing so he invited me over to his house. Mags and Sorcha were floored that I was with him. I called over to his house at 4:15. I rang the doorbell and he arrived out wearing blue jeans, a grey t-shirt and a baseball cap on backwards. Fwoargh! His house was an absolute mess because his parents are away. He showed me around the gaff. His room is covered in medals and trophies, mostly for karate. We listened to CDs and danced in the living room and had an amazing snog. He's well able to hold a conversation and we talked for ages. He gave me a lift home and said he'd call me when my phone number comes through the wash, but serious doubts if it's going to be legible. [*When it comes through the wash?! What? He must have told me that the piece of paper I'd written my number on was in his pocket and had 'accidentally' gone into the washing machine and I totally fell for it. Oh Jules! I feel I should mention that back in the day, I can't believe I just typed those words, but back then, 20 flippin' years ago, the guy always took the girl's phone number and we waited for him to call. We didn't have mobile phones, remember. So it was never the other way around like is the norm these days for a girl to initiate a call or a text message. We had to endure the big, long wait and it came through a message from your mum or dad as to whether he was on the phone or he had called while you were out and only then would we dial his number. How we had the patience to endure it, I'll never know.*] If he didn't call, I wouldn't be totally devastated. I couldn't be bothered sellotaping myself to the phone or getting obsessed with guys anymore. If he calls, he calls. He can't run away anyway because I'll see him every Saturday in the Bull & Bear. If my number doesn't come through the wash, he could look me up in the phone book and I also remembered that he has my two LL Cool J CDs and my phone number is written on the inside covers. I still can't believe I snogged Peter Andre's long-lost twin! Mum was nearly out buying her hat. She was saying that our kids will be gorgeous with dark skin and big brown eyes. If he wants me he can come and get me.

Plus tard – I've just read back this entry and it sort of sounds like I'm not into Robbie, well I so am but I'm just not getting unnecessarily worked up about it. He's a babe and a half, so I figure if I become really into him it could be nipped in the bud. I'll have to have a chillectomy and just go with the flow.

## 18 March 1996

A week has passed and there were no calls. I went to the Bull & Bear last night and he was there, looking fine. So I stalled around the DJ box and waited for him to come into my web. I was chatting to Caroline and then I saw him and decided I'd casually stroll by him. He was talking to one of his friends so I tapped him on the shoulder and he turned around and said 'Oh my God, how's it going?' and I said 'Fine, thanks' and he then abruptly turned his back on me and continued his conversation with his friend, while I stood there like a vegetable. I mean what's the story? I was with him last weekend, he invites me up to the gaff, we get on really well and then he doesn't even acknowledge me a week later?! I'm so depressed. The other thing is that he still has my CDs, I hope he's not thinking of keeping them 'cos that ain't going to happen. Men have such small brains! Oh well there's plenty more fish in the freezer!

## *20 March 1996*

I got my CDs back! Mags and I drove over to his gaff and I called in to pick them up. He took ages to get to the door and when he did answer all I could see was this brown eye peeping out. He had been in bed and he was only wearing a pair of Levi's. God he looked so fine! I think I totally caught him off-guard. No way was he expecting to see me at his door! I am the woman! I took the CDs and said 'See ya!' and strolled off. He was treading on some seriously thin ice messing with me! I had a cool speech planned that I was going to say but I didn't get the opportunity. The plan was that he opens his front door and sees me (this is obviously a dream so I'm looking stunningly attractive, good hair day, perfect make-up, tanned and I have a size 10 white Calvin Klein dress on). Anyway, I say 'I'm here to get my CDs' and he says 'Sure c'mon in, I'll get them ... So how are you?' Then I say 'Yeah, as if you care'. Then he replies 'What do you mean?' and I say 'Look Robbie, you've made enough of a fool out of me as it is, so just quit while you're ahead.' Gobsmacked at my feminine power, he says 'I don't understand'. I reply 'Do I have to spell it out for you? Do you even go to school? If you remember I was with you two weeks ago and we got on really well and then one week later I say hi to you and you don't even acknowledge me! I just think you made a complete fool out of me in front of all my friends. You're a sleaze, Robbie. I just can't believe I got stuck in your web. You've made a major mistake messing with me. Hell hath no fury like a woman scorned!' And then I head for the front door and stop, flick my hair and look back and say 'Especially me.' Then I jump into my bright yellow convertible Fiat Punto and speed away into the night. Then he sends me endless roses and sorry letters and after he pledges his undying love for me on national TV I decide that maybe he is worth taking back. So I hire him as my servant to carry my shopping bags!

I'm going through all stages of my closure. 1) Denial. I'm dreaming and I sure as hell better wake up soon. 2) Anger. I'm going to plunge my hand through his chest and rip out his still beating heart and hold it in front of his face so he can see how black it is before he dies! 3) Fear. What if I never get another man? (I don't think so!) 4) Acceptance. I am so over him, I've lapped him twice! That's it. Decision made. I'm not getting attached anymore. It's Girl Power in full effect from now on. It's seriously erase, replace, embrace, new face. Mr Right is out there somewhere and I'm not going to find him until I'm about 21 and if they want me they can come and get me. I'm so over him! I have CLOSURE! (I know I'm lying to myself, but I'll find someone new to fancy soon. I always do! I have a new chat up line ready 'Hey there dynamite, can I light your fuse?' Let's see what results that gets!)

With the assistance of alcohol, clocking up the snogs became even easier. In order to get into the over-18s discos, I needed a fake ID. So I got an application form for a student card, filled it out in cartridge pen and smiled sweetly while I got the school secretary to stamp it. Then with the Houdini magic of my ink eraser pen, I wiped out all the details on the form and changed them in biro so I had now magically aged three years and was of legal drinking age. I sent off the form and a few weeks later my legit student card arrived in the post and I was ready for my first taste of booze. I remember the anticipation of what it was going to feel like to be drunk. I had no idea what to expect. I nervously took a sip from a bottle of Bud and because I didn't know it would be so foamy, it dribbled down my chin (I seem to have done a lot of dribbling back in those days). By the time I was halfway through the bottle, I was feeling tipsy. What is this new magical feeling? It's like everything is just a little bit numb and I can't wipe the satisfied-with-life smile off my face.

My inhibitions flew out the window and like a mating ritual you'd see on a David Attenborough programme, I was breaking it down on the dance floor with my fellow pissed-up girlfriends like we were the actual Spice Girls on stage at a sold-out Wembley. Competition was fierce amongst all the girls in my class as you'd be fully in fear of not having a snog to report back about on Monday morning in school. So in order to ensure we got a result, the fashion stakes were upped. At this stage I had embraced my figure. I was slim and sexy and I was not afraid to show it. I had two hot-to-trot outfits that I wore and in them I was guaranteed to pull. One was a white belly-top t-shirt with the Calvin Klein logo on it. I would team this with black parallel trousers and the *pièce de résistance* was a pair of men's Calvin Klein boxers, which I would wear so the white CK elastic waistband was on view peeping out from the top of my trousers. That look was the essence of cool at the time and I thought I was the dog's conkers as I strutted around, leaving no one under any illusion as to what underwear I had on. (Men's jocks, Jules, you were wearing men's jocks! How did you think this was sexy?) My other sure-fire outfit quite literally spelled out that I was up for it. It was a belly-top t-shirt that had a picture of Little Miss Naughty from *Mr Men* on the front of it and I wore it with a black mini-skirt. Certified snogs were on the cards any time I wore either of these threads.

I remember that an entire night out on the piss back then cost £15. That would include bus fare, entry into the club, cloakroom, two bottles of Ritz cider (that's all we needed to get fish-faced) and a taxi home. Thankfully, we only ever got tipsy in those days, there weren't any passed-out people or vomiting; that would all come in later years when we hit the spirits. Sometimes we'd snog several people in one night and it's no wonder I was down at the doctor's on a regular basis getting antibiotics for tonsillitis. We were all the same though, it was a tsunami of hormones in the club as 300 15- and 16-year-olds experimented with each other's mouths and bodies. The night would start with keeping your eyes peeled for babes while standing in the jam-packed queue to get in the door. Then you'd flash your fake ID at the bouncer and stroll into the club. The next most important manoeuvre was a confident strut around the edge of the dance floor to the bathroom to check your face as God only knows what could have happened to your make-up and hair between the front door and bathroom. Then it was up to the bar to order a drink, all the while being in full Navy SEAL mode, scanning the club for potential hotties. Once your target was engaged, a lock-on was enforced through lots of flirty eye contact, hair flicking and 'I'm so not checking you out but I totally am' expressions on your face.

We got so good at the mating rituals we were able to predict when the slow set was going to start and we would have already nipped out to the toilets to fix our sweaty faces and plaster on more lipstick in the hope of smearing someone else's lips with it. Then, like something from a pass-the-parcel game at a kids' party, the dance music would come to an abrupt halt and a soppy, slow love song would begin playing. Everyone would commence using their best drama skills to show that they weren't desperate for a snog and would walk as slowly as possible off the dance floor in the hope of being approached and asked to dance. Sometimes the boys would send their friends over to ask 'Will you shift my friend?' and then point over to the requester while he stood there looking like a cheesy model from a fashion catalogue, pretending to check the time on his watch. This was great as you didn't have to refuse them directly if you didn't like the look of them. But if he was cheeky, the friend would then say, 'Well, will you shift me then?' Sometimes refusal lines would have to be rolled out, my favourite being, 'I'm sorry, I'm saving myself for Brad Pitt.'

Back in school, first thing on Monday morning, I'd whip out my homework notebook to log who now loved who. I went through numerous bottles of Tipp-Ex updating the weekly love profiles on the inside cover.

'Right. Sorcha, who did you snog again?'

'Philip, Michael and Cian.'

'Okay, so who am I putting down in the love corner?'

'Niall O'Brien.'

'But you didn't snog him.'

'Yeah I know, but I walked past him and I could smell his Fahrenheit aftershave and it was just divine plus he had a blue Ralph Lauren shirt on, so now I'm totally in love with him and he's my target for next week.'

'Nice one! Sorcha loves Niall.'

I put a huge amount of creative effort into my homework notebooks. They rarely contained any actual information about what homework I was supposed to be doing. They were just filled with notes from the girls who were either enraptured by a boy, heartbroken or moaning about their 'famine', which is what we used to call the length of time since our last snog.

*1995*

Hiya Jules,

How's life? Mine's shit. I'm living for Bective disco on Saturday. I swear to God I am not coming out of that place unsnogged. I'd even snog Harry the bouncer if it came to it – well maybe not. I'm not that desperate yet. I think I might go for a new record on Saturday – but it depends on how I feel or how trolloxed I am! Anyway, any decent looking bloke is not getting out of that place unsnogged!!! I'm sure you'll help me with that task! We're gonna have a feast not a famine! I LOVE _____
(I'll fill this in on Monday).

C-Ya, Luv, Sorcha xxx

## 1996

DJ Jules,

How are ya? Well I'm totally depressed, confused, in love and above all knackered. Life is so hard. The only thing that keeps me going is snogging and I'm a bit low on that at the moment. Right now I'd just like to know where I stand. I've got a really annoying tickly cough. Oh God I want him so badly! When I think of all the other people I fancied I'm like yeah right!

Anyway I'm too tired to write anymore so I'll say ciao, love Yvette xoxoxo

Well, I'll tell you one big thing I've learned from looking back on all of this is that there is no way I am sending my future kids to a single-sex school. I absolutely believe that because we were only around girls all day long and had no opportunity to interact with boys properly, apart from chowing down on their faces every weekend, that's why we became absolutely obsessed with them, because they were aliens to us. Can you imagine what we would have been like if we'd had mobile phones?! We only had landlines back then and all the time you'd be depending on the guy calling the house and then you'd have to take the phone into a press under the stairs to talk to him so nobody could hear your conversations. If I'd had a mobile phone, I would have been lethal, bombarding the boys with text messages. The best I could rely on was writing them letters, which I would post to their schools and God only knows how many priests and principals infiltrated and read them before they reached their intended recipient. I'd say they had some laugh in the staff room at break-time recounting my correspondence with the boys. Can you imagine them? 'Oh! It's another letter from Jules! This time it's for Andrew O'Keefe. She must have moved on from Henry Wilkinson. Let's see what she has to say to this poor chap!'

### 27 January 1996

Okay let's roll out the red carpet, the bells are ringing ... I am in love! Today I got my long-awaited letter from Andrew. I was so convinced he wasn't going to write back or that he didn't get my letter. For the past two weeks I've been strip searching the letterbox and just when I'd given up all hope and my arm was black and blue, I found a letter written in typically scrawly, boyish writing staring back at me. I bounded up the driveway shrieking like a hyena. His letter is so male, it's pathetic, but it's the thought that counts. I wouldn't have cared if he had only written two words in Swahili. It's so typically male, macho man, he was obviously taken aback by my letter, which I must admit was brilliant. I am dying to get my photos developed because he is in about 90 of them. I can't wait to write to him again. How shall I bear such happiness?

## 30 January 1996

I sent letter number two to Andrew today. It was four pages long. I asked him about 50 million questions in it so he'd have stuff to write back about. Valentine's Day is in 15 days' time, but Andrew will be on mid-term so he won't be in school and I don't have his home address! Dilemma! I suppose I'll just have to send a card to his school and wait until he goes back to get it.

## 14 February 1996

Well Andrew is out the window! I got no Valentine's card so he must really care. Not! I didn't get a reply to letter number two yet either. I'm praying that I can go out tomorrow night. I need a new man. My famine is way too long!

## 24 February 1996

I got letter number two from Andrew today. Two weeks ago I would have been having an eppo but I'm so not at the mo. He said he'd be 'honoured to be my Valentine' and he apologised for not sending me a card. Whatever. I haven't seen him for two months so I've totally gone off him. His letter was better than the first one, but it's still full of spelling mistakes, major turn-off and that just shows that he's obviously really immature. Why can't I find a man who can keep up with me on the witty writing front? He said he wants my phone number. I'm contemplating whether or not to write back to him. I certainly don't fancy him as much as I used to, but I figure maybe it's better to have him in reserve than not to? I think I'll write him a short letter. It'll be fun to keep in contact.

### 2 March 1996

I wrote a letter back to Andrew but I don't think I'll bother sending it. I've shown his letter to loads of people and they all think he has a single-digit IQ. I'm not associating myself with some intellectually challenged pleb! He's a total bimbo and I can't even be bothered writing back to him as friends if he can't even write back in Ladybird English. Smell ya later Andrew. Done. Over it.

I was just so desperate for a boy to love me and tell me I was beautiful. How ridiculous, looking back. And these coveted boys were just teenage morons with Lynx deodorant on their armpits, Pamela Anderson posters on their walls and wanking themselves around the cock day and night. Yet I was convinced that each one I snogged was my future husband.

One thing I did do, and I regret, was to lose my virginity when I was 16. Everyone has a chapter that should remain unwritten and this is mine. I did the deed purely because I thought my peers would think I was a total legend, but their reaction was in fact the opposite. I wrote to one of my best friends, Fiona, who was spending the summer in France and I told her all about how I had 'done it'. I thought I was the business. Fiona wrote back and told me

> Jules, I am completely gobsmacked by your news. I can't believe that my friend who I have known since she was five years old is now, how should I put it? Not a little girl anymore. I'm in shock. But I have to say, Jules, we are going to have some serious words when I get home. I know we all talk about sex all the time, but wasn't it like an unspoken rule that we all knew it was such a serious thing that we weren't ever going to actually do it until we were adults? I mean you could get pregnant

and have to leave school and what would we all do then?! Well you've done it now, so there's no taking it back unfortunately.

An unspoken rule?! I wasn't aware of this! I thought it was a goal we all had. What a plonker. When I didn't get the reaction from my close friends that I expected, I was fearful that news was going to get around about it and I would be considered a slut. So I told all the girls that it was a huge mistake and they all promised to keep their lips zipped and I swore I'd keep my knickers zipped in future and we would say no more about it. I was utterly ashamed of my antics and felt so small I could have sat on the edge of a Rizla paper with my legs dangling off. So I decided to pretend it never happened and convinced myself that, like a cherry tree reblossoms each season, I was a born-again virgin. That was, until Mum found out about it. I left the letter Fiona had written to me telling me of her perturbedness at my virginal loss out on my desk in plain sight and Mum saw it. Thankfully, her reaction was to have a compassionate chat with me about it and I broke down crying. Mum is always great in these situations. Some parents would shout and scream at you, but Mum helped me through it with love and empathy. This was a landmark shift in my life. Lessons were learned and, thankfully, a new peak of maturity was reached because of it.

*August 1995. Age: 16.*

'Hi Jules'

'Hi!'

'How's it going?'

'Fine. I'm tired.'

'Do you like going back to school?'

'Yeah, because I want to see everybody, but not the sitting in the class aspect of things.'

'Why did you take down your Manchester United posters?'

''Cos it's the new me. Just the new me. I've turned over a new leaf, a new branch, a new tree.'

'What sort of tree would you be?'

'Em ... An oak tree because it grows old and mature, I don't know! It's the new intellectual, mature, sophisticated me. I was a little acorn and now I'm going to be an oak tree.'

'What about boys?'

'What about them? They're thick. A waste of time.'

'How about Barry?'

'Oh God! He'll grow up some day I suppose!'

'Do you like yourself?'

'I don't know. I like the new me, ya know? Not doing everything to impress others.'

'Plans for the year?'

'Study in school. There's not going to be much more to my life, is there?'

'What do you think of Mike and me?'

'Well, what do you mean, on what front like? (avoids question) I like ya! I have to get dressed.'

'And we love you too Jules.'

As part of the new mature me who was taking responsibility for her life, I got a job in McDonald's so I could earn money to buy clothes and my weekly *Smash Hits* magazine instead of having to beg Mum all the time for things. I thought it would be great. Free Maccy D's for lunch every day! But it wasn't until I got behind the counter and started prepping the food that I found out how completely turned off by it I was. My job was to dress the burgers. I was lightning-fast at it and in addition to squirting ketchup on patties every morning, I would wheel out the vat of white lard and scoop it into the fryers to make the chips. It was disgusting when you saw it in solid form. For the first few days at break-time, I had my favourite quarter-pounder and fries, but a few mornings of lard duty and I quickly switched to going to the local shop for a sandwich. Thank God this happened as I could have ended up piling on the pounds if I'd been eating that grease-laden grub every day.

At this point in my life, I was still slim. I ate pretty much whatever I wanted and my size was just normal. I got lots of exercise in school between PE and playing basketball, hockey and tennis four days a week. I was elected sports secretary as I was so involved in all things sporty, so at least I was burning off serious calories to counteract my sweet and savoury tooth. We didn't have a tuck shop or vending machines in school and the local shop was a 15-minute walk away, so when it came to forming our mini-company for a transition year assignment and I was tasked with the position of production manager, I knew exactly what we'd be selling: my favourite, jam doughnuts. We bought them in bulk from the local bakery and whacked on a 200% profit margin and sold them in the canteen at lunchtime. We were creaming it in with our jammy enterprise and I was scoffing them like an unchaperoned child at a birthday party. Our favourite challenge, which was merely an excuse to eat a multitude of them, was to try and eat a doughnut without licking your lips. 'Aaaah! I saw that! You defo licked them!' 'Okay, okay, hang on, let me finish this one and we'll start again. I'll do it this time!' They were great days back then, when I could eat what I wanted with no chubby consequences.

My mad snogging nights out had calmed down at that stage. I still desperately wanted a boyfriend. And I finally got one when I bumped into the newly transformed Gordon, Daniel's (my first kiss) best friend. Gone was his *Wayne's World* hair. He had cut it short and shaved down his beard into a goatee. How had I never noticed his good looks before this? He now looked super-hot. He'd cracked out of his shy shell and was now much more confident and talkative. Flirting began and when he told me he'd always had a crush on me, I was ecstatic and immediately threw the lips on him.

*9 February 1996. Age: 16 and ½.*

'Well, Jules, you asked for this interview. What have you got to say for yourself?'

'About what? You're meant to ask the questions!'

'What do you think of Gordon?'

'Two weeks, four days now. He's a babe. Nobody knows him except me. He is my Mr Darcy in the flesh. He puts on a real macho image, but he's a softy underneath.'

'Do you think you'll marry him?'

'Duuuuuh! What a stupid question! I only have to add "ins" onto my surname so it's a bit of a sign, I reckon.'

'Where do you see yourself in a couple of years?'

'Finished school and on my way to becoming a billionaire.'

'What about your love life?'

'Well, I'll still be going out with Gordon. I'd say we'll get married at 26 – 'cos I'll have to pursue my career without the hassles of being tied down.'

'Do you think he can wait that long?'

'He'll wait if I tell him to. I've got him wrapped around my little finger.'

'Do you not think that the man should have the dominant role?'

'Well, eh! I never said that … It's not a case of roles. I mean we're both in control to some extent, it's just that I have him at my feet.'

'Why, if that's the case, don't I get to meet him?'

'You can meet him at the wedding reception.'

'How would you describe yourself?'

'Me? Smooth, suave, sophisticated.'

'Favourite TV and radio?'

'*Bottom* No. 1 of course. *Pride and Prejudice*. *X-Files*. *Ab Fab* and *The Young Ones*.'

'Do you think we have a good mother–daughter relationship?'

'Yeah! You're a nice person and if you want to give me money at any time – you're looking young and unwrinkley and your nails and hair are looking great! The acupuncture is having a great effect on you!'

'Would you like acupuncture?'

'Well, if I get the results you get then I'd love it! Yeah, apparently I'm under stress.'

'What stress?'

'Don't know really. Well actually it was just that Gary fellow who brought me on a date and then never called me again. Absolute twat. I'm alright with Gordon now.'

'Do you have a final word before we finish?' (Farts at this point. Then laughs and thinks she's charming.)

'I've got a really spotty back – can acupuncture help spotty backs?'

When Valentine's Day rolled around I was really excited. This was the first time I was going to have a boyfriend for Cupid's big day. Gordon and I had only been going out for three weeks, but I was looking forward to him showering me with gifts. When a big basket of red and white carnations with a 'Kiss Me' teddy bear arrived at the front door, I was hysterical. I phoned Gordon to thank him, but he told me he didn't send them. 'Well, if you didn't send them, who the bloody hell did?' I wondered. I later found out that it was Terry, Gordon's best friend, who apparently had a crush on me. What a weirdo. Gordon hadn't gotten me anything for Valentine's Day. Cheers! It lasted a mere week after that before it went pear-shaped and it was all over, but Terry obviously saw this as an available opening and when I received an anonymous letter in the post, I knew it was from him. I don't have the letter to relay exactly what it said because I have since burned it, but it was filled with lewd descriptions and drawings of what he wanted to do to me and as a token of his undying affection for me he'd also included a present of some of his pubes in the envelope. Yes, pubes. I wanted to vomit everywhere when I opened it. It was so creepy and freaked me out so much I took it to the Gardaí, who told me that if I received another one not to open it and then they could fingerprint it. Thinking back though, it had actual DNA evidence in it thanks to his hairy gift, but I suppose what are they going to arrest him for? Being an ominous perv? Thankfully, I didn't receive any more vile correspondence but I burned the hairy letter as I couldn't bear to have it in the house. I was so done with boys at that point. I was just sick of all the drama and the intensity of the soap opera antics. I decided to concentrate entirely on working on my portfolio to secure my place in art college.

*29 March 1996. Age: 16 and ½.*

Mock Interview Assessment

Very well presented. Very friendly. Relaxed. Amiable. Excellent CV and portfolio very good. Has an obvious talent for her chosen career. Sure it suits her well. Talks too fast – she knows this and should try and work on it. Has a habit of looking down now and again and should improve eye contact. Hands move a lot. Shoulders shrugged a little – improve the posture. Should consider the summer job as a chance to commence practical work in her chosen environment?

Initially I had no clue what I wanted to do in college. I still had little interest in school work apart from Art and English. Everything else was a snore and I wondered when in my life I was ever going to use Pythagoras' theorem or when were the details of the complex insides of a piece of seaweed or an earthworm ever going to be required while I was off shopping in Beverly Hills seven days a week? They have never even come up in a table quiz since I left school. Has anyone ever actually seen an oxbow lake?

They really taught us such a load of bollocks, didn't they? We should have been learning life skills instead. Things like case studies of moral dilemmas, how to change a car tyre, public speaking and nutrition classes. At least we could have put those into practice in everyday life instead of $x + y =$ the square root of who the feck cares? We attended lots of college open days to see the courses on offer. I only went as it meant a day off school, but when I walked into the make-up room in Dun Laoghaire College of Art and Design, my heart flipped. There were 20 white desks, each with a mirror surrounded by multiple lightbulbs around the edge, just like in the movies. 'Sorry, what's this course in here?' I eagerly enquired. 'Special FX make-up for television, film and theatre,' I was told. Sign me up. I am loving this! A make-up artist. What a cool job! I worked night and day on my portfolio, which would be graded and added to my Leaving Cert exam points in addition to an interview to get in as there were only 20 places on the course. I am going to be one of those 20, I told myself. Yes I am! Jules Coll – make-up artist to the stars. Yeah baby! I could do make-up in Hollywood and fall in love with Johnny Depp! Feckin' deadly! This is me, this is so me.

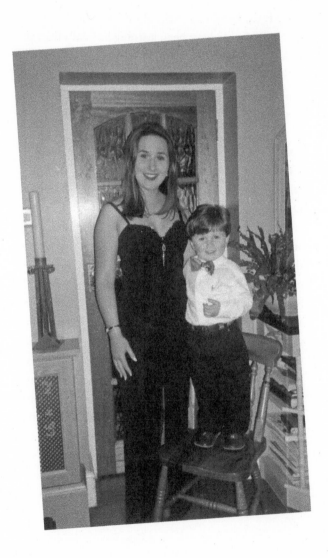

# 4

## *Labour Pains*

*June 1996. Age: Nearly 17.*

Your bank account is empty. You have an insatiable appetite for money. Always needing more no matter how much you get. I had to fork out £15 for the job you did on the table and bench. You painted OVER the spiders and their webs and left four big brown patches on Mike's precious grass. I had to go on a message and when I got back you met me at the front door moaning and whining about how you couldn't get the stains off your arms, legs, face and hands even though you had been scrubbing yourself for hours. It turned out that instead of white spirits you'd been using Benlate – a fungicide for black spot on roses. What a plonker! Anyway I told you to look on the bright side – at least you've no chance of getting black spot or mildew (or more painting jobs for that matter – we won't mention the front wall). I'd stick to face painting if I were you.

*W*hat do you say when you're aged 17, strolling down Grafton Street on a sunny Sunday afternoon, after a lovely lunch with your parents, and your 45-year-old mum casually says, 'Oh yes, I have to pop into the pharmacy to get a pregnancy test.' 'To get a WHAT?' I exclaimed. 'A pregnancy test,' she confirmed. 'What?! For me?! I told you I've been like extra virgin olive oil! I haven't slept with anyone I swear!' I retorted. 'I know, I know. It's for me,' she replied. 'For YOU?! Mum! This is mental! Are you having a giraffe?!' I almost shouted. 'Not a giraffe, but perhaps a baby,' she quipped.

I was gobsmacked, initially just at the thought that Mum and Dad were still doing it. *Ewww!* But then at the realisation that Mum was actually serious. She was so casual about it. I think it must be due to the fact that she too was in as much shock as I was. The pregnancy test result was positive. Dad promptly went paler than a snowman with anaemia and passed out on their bed. Barry and I couldn't believe it either. When the initial consternation settled and the bombshell was defused, we were all actually overjoyed. A baby! A new member of the family. Mum and Dad were both 45 so this was to be a 'geriatric pregnancy', and we slagged Mum endlessly over this term. I was 17 and Barry was 15, both of us nearly finished with school. Just when they thought all the school runs and exams were coming to an end, groundhog day clocked in and it was a case of 'return to Go, do not collect £200, get ready for 18 more years of parent–teacher meetings and homework.'

Mum's pregnancy was fascinating. I learned so much as we became obsessed with all things childbirth and the only thing we watched on TV was baby programmes. It was 15 years since Mum had delivered Barry, so she needed a full refresher course. I couldn't wait to have a little bundle of joy in the house so I could dress him or her in cute little outfits. I have always been the maternal type and caring for a child is something that still to this day fills me with overwhelming joy. As Mum's bump grew, so did my family's excitement. I remember lying in bed late one night when the bump was the size of a beach-ball and hearing Mum gently say from her bedroom, 'Jules?' and I knew just by the tone of her voice that it was baby arrival time. I bounded out of the bed and the four of us headed to the hospital, ecstatic to meet the newest Coll. Gavin was born on 12 January 1997 weighing nine pounds 13 ounces, after an emergency C-section following 24 hours of intense labour. Thankfully he was fine and he looked like a gorgeous little human prune when he came out and the nurse wrapped him in a blue blanket. I was instantly in love. 'You are not getting a look in,' I told Mum. 'This is going to be the easiest child-rearing ever because I am going to change all his nappies and put Sudocrem on his teeny little willy and give him baths and bottles and train him to be a DJ and bring him to the zoo!' Mum laughed and continued clicking the magic morphine button as she lay in her hospital bed.

Gavin was probably the most fussed-over baby in the country. He had four parents as we were all devoted to looking after him, making him laugh and stimulating him educationally, convinced he was going to be the next president of Ireland. By the time he was two, he was like a mini-adult with a gigantic vocabulary. He had the voice of a toddler but chatted away like a little old man. He was gas! His favourite thing to do was sit on my bed and listen to my music. He quickly picked up the words and some dance moves to 'Horny' by Mousse T., which was a hugely popular song at the time and he'd sing the lyrics, 'I'm horny! Horny! Horny! Horny!', at the top of his lungs in the supermarket while sitting in the trolley. I'd be laughing my head off as the proudest sister in the world. People would stare and judge and I'd think, 'Ah feck off, ya dry shite. It's his favourite song! He picked it! And it's No. 1 in the charts right now so you'd wanna start listening to the radio, ya boring sod.' I also noticed, when he wasn't singing 'Horny', the looks I'd get from some people who would look down on me seeing that I was obviously a teenager and thinking Gavin was my child and assuming Mum was the granny. They would hold open doors and let people pass and then see me with the buggy and let go of the door and swing it back in my face. This happened on several occasions and I recall being shocked at how I was treated just because I was a young person pushing a pram that contained my little brother. But who cares if it had been my son, who are you to judge, you old barnacle? Go back and live with the dinosaurs where you belong! I should have hailed a taxi and said, 'A one-way fare to Jurassic Park, please,' and kicked them into the back seat and slammed the door.

That September I left my cherished girlfriends in secondary school and moved for sixth year to the Institute of Education on Leeson Street in Dublin because they had an incredible art teacher. It was great because it was mixed. So if I wasn't in art class, I was either window-shopping on Grafton Street, drinking coffee in a café or hanging out with guys in St Stephen's Green Park. It didn't feel like school at all. I loved it.

After graduating school in June 1997, I started the make-up course in college, when Gavin was six months old. Oh yes, did I forget to mention that I got top marks for my portfolio, aced the interview and bagged myself one of the 20 coveted places on the course in Dun Laoghaire College of Art and Design? Well, it wasn't a big deal really. Sorry, what was that you said? 'How many people tried to get in?' Oh not that many, only a thousand. 'And you got a place? Wow!' Well, it was nothing really. 'Jules, your portfolio must have been incredible.' Ah I just threw a few bits together over a weekend really and they seemed to like it. 'That's amazing!' I'm amazing? Will ya stop, you're making me scarlet!

I had become so attached to little Gav that it pained me to leave him for eight hours a day. But at least the excitement of my new make-up kit, which came in a big toolbox, was there to distract me. The course was fantastic and we learned everything possible about make-up, wigs and special FX. College life was also great. Gone were the draconian days of secondary school, where the teachers would stop you in the corridor to check the length of your skirt and as they'd bend down to inspect the hem, you'd have to resist the urge to knee them in the face. College meant freedom. They treated us like adults and if you wanted to turn up for the classes and get a distinction, then you could. Or if you wanted to sit around on bean bags all day talking bollocks and fail, you could do that too. The choice was yours. I loved my course so much I threw myself into it.

I did the same with the socialising. Student life meant we were all as broke as Lent on Paddy's Day, but we still found ways to go on the lash. Pre-drinking was the first obvious choice. We'd tank ourselves up in someone's gaff before getting the bus into town and then of course be compelled to swing around the poles on the bus shouting, 'Look at me, I'm Demi Moore in *Striptease*!' The next clever money-saving tactic was to bring a naggin of vodka with you in your handbag. Bouncers would check our bags as we went into nightclubs, so my remedy for this was to buy a really cheap handbag, cut a slit in the lining and hide the vodka bottle inside the lining material. Genius. Then I'd place all my usual crap like empty wallet, make-up, hair brush and chewing gum on top and display that to the bouncer and he was none the wiser. Once inside the club, we mastered the art of subtly whipping out the naggin, like we were wearing invisibility cloaks, and topping up our soft drinks so we could get absolutely national lampooned at minimum cost.

We rinsed the kegs a few nights a week. I was practically growing gills. And now that I was out drinking in the city centre, I discovered the Lamb of God ... kebabs.

As a younger teen going out on the lasharoo, I'd only have a couple of drinks and then stuff an entire packet of chewing gum into my mouth on the way home in the taxi in case I was greeted by Mum or Dad as I climbed in my bedroom window at 3 a.m. I didn't get any hangovers and I guess that's because it only took two drinks to get me langers, so my virile liver had no trouble at all processing that and I would wake up the next morning as fresh as a princess in Bel Air. It was only when the spirits were added to the guest list that my liver went straight to its union for talks and started pickling. I was now out getting properly pissed and this led to intense desires for anything salty and greasy at the end of a night. With a big happy head on me, I'd drag my knuckles across the floor of Abrakebabra and squint one eye to focus on the menu. 'Keebib 'n chiz 'n gallic fraz, plez. Tanks.' Why do they taste 50 million times more amazing when you're gee-eyed at three o'clock in the morning? I'd wake up the following noon and my breath would smell like Oscar the Grouch's bin juice and I'd look like the love child of one of Roald Dahl's witches and Freddie Krueger. With my student life now consumed by classes, boozing and recovering, I was getting as much exercise as a sloth on Valium. Uh oh.

The only part of my body that was getting any exercise was my tongue and not just from eating, from snogging.

Snog number: 55

Name: Alex —

College: DLCAD

Eyes: Brown

Hair: Dark brown

Looks: 9/10

Snogability: 10/10

*6 November 1997*

What a babe. The minute I walked into the room at the party he caught my beady eye. I've never seen him before in college. Apparently he's seen me loads of times. He knew the jacket I wear etc. Oh my God stalker! I love it! I got talking to him when I was coming down the stairs after I broke a nail and he was comforting me. I was chatting away to him for ages. He's doing the radio course and I was telling him I used to be on Pulse FM and we were chatting about the buzz you get going on the radio and doing gigs. He's 21, a nice mature man, just what the doctor ordered! His dream woman is Louise from Eternal apparently. When I asked him that he was supposed to say me. Well that backfired. He's so funny and chatty and he's a gentleman. I snogged him on the stairs and he's an amazing kisser. He bought me chips as we walked up to the phone box and I called a taxi and he waited with me for it. He said he's seen me around in college and has been eyeing me up for weeks. He knew I was dressed up as Dame Edna at the Hallowe'en party and everything. How have I never noticed his fine self before? I so fancy him. All the girls said there were mad jealous 'cos I got Alex. I saw him in the canteen at break-time the next day. There was loads of flirty eye contact but I would have had to have done an Anneka Rice over all the tables to go over to him 'cos the place was packed. This has to become my college relationship. He will be mine, oh yes, he will be mine!

*21 November 1997*

Oh I am so in love. I was in the canteen and Tara introduced me to the magical combo of chips and mayonnaise, it's unreal! It's probably really fattening but I don't care it's so yummy! So there I was drooling all over the plate and I saw Alex leaving so I decided to bite the bullet to go after him. (I left the chips and mayonnaise behind, that's how hot he is!) I caught him in the corridor. I wasn't nervous at all, he's so easy to talk to. Then on Tuesday I met him in the library. I was looking through the shelves and I saw these gorgeous little Maltesers-brown eyes looking through from the other side. He helped me find the book I was looking for. He's so cute. Later I was talking to him in the canteen and just as I was about to ask him if he was going out tonight some bimbo came over and said his tutor wanted to speak to him. What a stupid cow. Today he was up on the window sill putting up a speaker – his ass should come with a government health warning! It's been major smiles and positive vibes but I think we're both too shy to do anything about it.

Snog number: 56

Name: Colin —

Place: Belvo

College: UCD

Looks: 8/10

Snogability: 9/10

He was wearing: Blue shirt, cream chinos

I was wearing: Tiger print belly-top, black parallels

## 29 November 1997

Nice guy. Great snog. I found that I had no problem talking to guys on the night 'cos I kept thinking about Alex the whole time. Colin was bet into seeing me again and wanted my phone number. I told him there was a potential guy in college and he asked could he see me again if things didn't work out with me and Alex? So to fob him off I told him that I'd be in Belvo next Saturday (I won't). It's just typical that the one time I'm not interested I have someone bet after my phone number. I'm so mad into Alex. I could totally see myself marrying him. His brown eyes are dreamy.

## 8 December 1997

Well there have been no developments with the ol' Alex situation to date. I said hi to him in the canteen last Friday, if that counts. Hardly. I so never see him around. Only three days to the Christmas social and we are totally snogging the faces off each other then. Mags called in on Sunday. She went to Belvo and guess who she bumped into? Colin, the guy I was with in Belvo last weekend and she found out he was there looking for me. I was floored when she told me. What's the bets now that I have someone interested in me – finally – and now things will work out with Alex. I'm so annoyed 'cos Colin is really nice. I'd be well up for being with him again, but I'm so crazy into Alex.

## 11 December 1997

I was with Alex at the Christmas party. I was absolutely leeched on the night. But nothing was said at all about seeing each other again outside college or any story so I decided he was out the window. Smell ya later shy Alex. I ain't got time for your bullshit! So I decided that I was well up for a bit of Colin. Little did I know that it was going to be the best Belvo ever!

## 13 December 1997

I'm so in love! I have a boyfriend!!! And we're engaged! So actually I have a fiancé! Went to Belvo and saw Colin there. Nearly passed out, he's so hot! Danced over to him and chatted away. I was with him for the entire night. He asked me out, asked me to marry him and he's buying the house this week. He's gas! And so nice and such a gentleman and he's so bet into me! Alex is history! I'm sorry I'm not home right now. If it's Colin calling please press one. If it's Alex please hang up.

Surprise, surprise, I went out with Colin for five weeks and then found out he'd been doing the dirt on me the whole time and he was an absolute gigolo. Charming.

The summer of 1998 is when everything went quite literally pear-shaped. I reunited with all my best girlfriends from school and we took a trip to Ios, one of the Greek islands. The plan was to spend three months there on the razzle dazzle in the sun. 'Yeah, we'll get some sort of shitty jobs when we run out of money, it'll be grand!' we thought. Fifteen of us trekked over and managed to find ourselves a cheap kip to live in for £3 each a night. All we had was a bed each that a prisoner would consider luxurious and a bedside locker. We pulled a MacGyver and made wardrobes for ourselves by opening out black bags and putting them on the filthy floor under our beds and laying out our skimpy holiday clothes on them. We all shared one shower and it was quite simply chaos. We loved it! Once the sunshine hit our transparent Irish skin, we were on the bus to banterland and going wild. There were loads of other Irish people there and the entire island was in party mode 24 hours a day. It was bonkers craic and we lapped it up.

Doing everything on the cheapo, we figured out that the best value bottles of wine were the ones that came in gallon-sized bottles. Dionysus was our main vino of choice. It tasted like rat's piss. We chugged it back and drank all the free promotional shots that they offered to entice you into clubs. Once they were consumed, we were out the door and heading into the adjacent club to avail of their freebies. Our main source of food was certainly not the internationally famous healthy Greek salad. Instead, we gravitated towards the Greek specialty that is a souvlaki, which is essentially a fluffy pitta bread filled with chips, meat (what type I have no idea and to be honest, I don't want to know!), onions and tzatziki, which is a magical creamy sauce that tasted like unicorn's jizz.

We sunbathed during the day and drank and danced on tables all night. When cash started running low, some of us faced the reality of looking for jobs. I managed to bag a waitress job in a pizza restaurant that was paying £1 an hour, which was the going rate. I stood in the restaurant, pissed off and sulking as I watched all the drunkards singing as they staggered through the streets. After two hours, when not one customer had entered the restaurant, I took off my apron, threw it over my shoulder and went to join all my mates out on the lash. Mum and Dad had given me a credit card for 'emergencies'. Well, having to pay my weekly rent and buy souvlakis and wine to feed and hydrate myself would be classed as a code red, wouldn't it? I started using the credit card to withdraw the odd £20 from the ATM, which would keep me going for a good few days, all the while thinking, 'It's

grand, I'll pay Mum and Dad back when I get home.
I'd rather do that than stand in that shite-hole pizzeria
staring at the floor like a fuckwit for £1 an hour. I
am so way better than that and I'm sure if Mum and
Dad could see such an abysmal working environment,
they'd be telling me to quit the job and just live it up,
wouldn't they?' No they wouldn't, Jules, you absolute
brat. After that, I considered myself to just be on one
big, long summer holiday with sand in my hair, sun on
my skin, wine in my belly and a big happy smile on my
freckly Irish face.

Of course, I kept a diary of the holiday, mostly so I
could recollect it when I came home as we were all
in the business of annihilating as many brain cells as
possible, so keeping an account of our Ios antics was
absolutely necessary. Whenever I was sober enough,
I would jot down what had happened the previous
night. Here's an account of a typical night in insane
Ios.

### 20 June 1998

Drank a bottle of crème de menthe mixed
with vodka before we went out. Took hilarious
photos of the lads after we turned them into
transvestites. I did their make-up and Caroline
dressed them. Staggered down to the square.
Drank warm Amstel sitting on the wall.

Sorcha and I snog two Australians. Danced on the tables in Sweet Irish Dream. Sorcha got a hickey on her leg. Ugly Swedish guy flashes his shorn scrotum to us as we walk by. Pointed and laughed. Got free cocktails and shots in Orgasm bar. Stumbled around the square for ages. Got Calippos and ice-cream. Laura snogged a Canadian. Savaged souvlakis in some rancid diner. Got flashed by two Brits who were on the phone to their mum telling her what a great time they're having. Went to bed fully clothed. Next day, we are all in a heap. I have the trots, they are green from the crème de menthe. Sorcha hasn't shat for seven days.

Eight weeks into my Greek adventure I got an email from Mum telling me that they'd received the Visa statement and that I had racked up a £300 bill. My eyes were out on stalks when I read it. Shiiiiit! How could I present a case to defend myself? I knew this was coming. What was my £300 emergency? The only real emergency that had taken place was when I split my chin open trying to get out of the pool while drunk. There was no doctor on the tiny island, so the girls brought me to the local vet to get it sewn up. He switched from spaying cats in the winter to looking after pissed-up humans for the summer and made a fortune doing it as us drunkards were so injury-prone. He even had a nice little scam going on where you could go to him and get your eyebrow or bellybutton pierced for free and he would claim on your medical insurance that he'd treated you for some other ailment, like a broken arm or leg. All you had to do was sign a form. So after two months of debauchery, I was ordered by Mum and Dad to get my drunk ass home to Ireland as I had obviously lost the run of myself. Tail between my legs and antiseptic cream on my bellybutton ring, I said goodbye to Ios and flew back to Dublin ready to promise my parents that I'd pay them back every cent of the £300 I had blown on my epic summer of insanity in Greece.

### *Summer of 1998. Age: 18/19.*

I'd say it was an experience. You obviously went wild and lived in squalor. The Visa card was your only means of survival and in the end I had to write to you by email and tell you to come home. We couldn't get over the amount of weight you'd put on in the two months. Obviously all the booze. We were glad to see you home safely. I certainly missed you around the place with just 'Three men and a little lady' in the house. No real steady boyfriend. Although you've been with all the DJs in Pulse FM and snogged half of Dublin. I've been at you to lose weight. You don't like hearing it but at the moment your weight is out of control. It's a shame to see someone so attractive lost in blubber. Hopefully you'll see the light before it's too late.

At this point, I would have weighed around 12 stone. I knew I had piled on the pounds, but I was choosing to ignore it. I could see it in the mirror but all the while I was telling myself, 'It's not that bad. You can start a diet on Monday and knock it off in no time. It'll be graaaaand.' It saddens me to read of Mum and Dad's shock at seeing me roll into the airport arrivals hall and suddenly see that I had puffed up and that it was very obvious. When it's happening to your own body, you don't notice it as much because it's such a slow process. It's not until you see an old photo or video of yourself that it hits home as to the extent of the difference.

Mum did gently broach the subject of my weight, but whenever the topic was mentioned, because it was such a sensitive issue for me, I immediately went full armadillo and went on the defence. I would say, 'I know! I am! I already have the diet planned. I know what I'm doing. I don't need any help. It's grand. Stop harping on about it!' and I'd leave the room. There are two types of people in this world when it comes to reacting after a conversation like that. One type storms off and sits on their bed and thinks to themselves, 'I'll show you! You think my weight's out of control and I can't get it back on track? Well just you wait and see me do it. You think I can't, but oh yes I can! I'll show you!' And then there's me. I was so incredibly defensive that I'd think to myself, 'If I start that diet tomorrow, she's gonna think that I did it because of what she said and when the weight falls off it'll be all, "Aren't you glad I encouraged you to do that now?" Ugh. I'll do it off my own bat, thanks very much! It's my body and my diet and I'll do it my way in my own time, not because you advised me to.' Again, deep down this was just another excuse to stay numb, in denial and stay stuck, because my mind had already gone into freefall about all of it. I was so panicked I had frozen, and it was easier to stay in La La Land thinking that I'd find an easy remedy to the problem and then everything would be back to normal again.

I completed my second year of college and throughout I was either on a diet for two weeks or on the piss eating taco fries. This is where the yo-yo rollercoaster of dieting began. When I finished my college course, I was under the impression that I'd don my cap and gown, whip the cap up in the air and watch it soar and by the time I'd look down to see it land, Steven Spielberg himself would be there in front of me on bended knee, holding out his cheque book and asking me to come and work for him. Sadly though, 1999, the year we graduated, was a really tough time in the TV and film industry and there was very little work for make-up artists. I ended up doing bits and pieces on small independent films, working for free just to gain experience and try to forge a good reputation for myself. I hit rock-bottom that November when I was working on an interior design TV show in Ardmore Studios in County Wicklow. I was there to make up the faces of the three presenters, one of whom was the biggest diva I've ever come across. How much of a diva was he? Well, one day he refused to let my make-up brushes touch his precious face until I drove to the nearest McDonald's and got him a Big Mac. Seriously. I did it just because it was the easiest option and I'd get my job done.

On one particular day, while I was busy trowelling foundation on faces, the show's producers were under huge time pressure to dress the sets so they looked like fancy bathrooms. When they ran out of copper mosaic tiles and didn't have time to source more, I was asked to step in and use my make-up skills to match up some other mosaic tiles in order to complete the set. And I did it because I'm all for everyone mucking in on a job, but I remember kneeling beside the toilet bowl painting tiny tiles and just thinking to myself, 'I am qualified to do make-up on the levels of *Star Trek*, what am I doing painting the back of a cistern?' I contemplated moving to London, where there would be loads of work, but

I couldn't leave my beloved baby brother Gavin, so I decided to wait impatiently for the right jobs to come around. Thankfully, Mum and Dad still provided a roof over my head and food in the fridge. What more could I need?

*14 October 2000. Age: 21.*

No work. Still waiting for the phone to ring with offers of make-up jobs. You spend your time hanging around the house watching TV and eating. You've piled on the weight and I don't know what to say or do to help you. It really upsets me to see you in such a rut. To see such a beautiful face being slowly distorted with excess fat. You need some direction and routine in your life and above all you need the love of a man – nothing on the horizon and my worry is that if you continue to eat for comfort, you will limit your chances of getting the pick of the crop. I just keep praying that you will one day wake up and see the light and get healthy. You are a lovely, lovely daughter and Mike and I want the best for you. Hopefully in 2001 you will find the direction and self-satisfaction you are looking for. This year brought a job as a receptionist in a recruitment agency. You hate it but at least it pays you a few bob to pay for your skiing holiday. Maybe next year you will change to something more rewarding.

No work. No money. No boyfriend. Well, actually I was in a relationship, an unhealthy relationship with food. This is when chocolate and I started dating seriously. I sat around the house all day watching TV and eating rings around myself. I found solace in a strong cup of tea and endless slices of toast with lashings of butter. In fairness though, I did help Mum out a lot around the house. She was under a lot of stress as she had a toddler and a building site in the back garden because Mum and Dad had decided to knock down our house and build a new one in its place. So at one point we were living in a half of what was the old house and I was sleeping in the dining room.

On the day that we were officially moving all of ten feet into the new gaff and the remains of the old house were being knocked down, I convinced Mum to let us graffiti the inside walls for the craic, seeing as it was all going to be pillaged to rubble anyway. Barry and I bought spray paint and began desecrating the place. 'What'll I write? Will I just write *fuck*?' I sniggered to Barry as we defaced every wall in sight and then took sledgehammers to the windows and took out all our stress and frustrations by plundering the place like two human wrecking balls. It was great fun and Mum just watched on and laughed at her two mad kids having a whale of a time. That was until the JCB arrived to begin demolition, along with all the neighbours who crowded around to see the destruction. The big claw of the heavy machinery plunged into the roof of the house and began tearing down the walls, thus revealing all the graffiti artwork with which Barry and I had littered the walls. Swear words, willies, anarchy symbols … the lot. Mum and Dad were mortified. Barry and I were in hysterics.

With little excitement in my boring life at this time, I had to seek it out for myself. I collected Barry from his school one day when he was doing his final year exams. The school car park was empty, so I got out of the car and let Barry into the driver's seat to teach him how to drive. He was having a great time just driving around in circles as we blared dance music. Then along came another car filled with a load of lads armed with cartons of eggs. They were celebrating the end of school and driving around egging anything in sight. They pelted my car with several eggs and I cracked. Like a level-ten detective, I noted the make, model, colour and registration of the car and thought to myself, in the voice of Samuel L. Jackson, 'You're going down, mothah fuckah!' I managed to get the eggs off my car after going through the car wash twice. The following day was revenge time. I bought a big plastic bucket and my shopping list from the local supermarket included dog food, sardines, two dozen eggs, garlic paste, mackerel, flour, buttermilk and anything else I spied on the shelves that smelled revolting. I mixed it all up in the bucket with a wooden spoon and secured it in the passenger seat of my car with the seatbelt. With all the windows down, as it smelled like the bog of eternal stench, I drove down to the school and found the Volkswagen Polo parked in the car park. I pulled up beside it. Filled with a phenomenal adrenaline rush, I proceeded to tip the entire contents of the bucket of gunge I'd whipped up all over egg-head's car and drove off at top speed, laughing my head off. Later on, Barry told me that when the guy came out to his car he got the fright of his life. Today's lesson: Don't mess with the Jules!

I found further excitement in expressing myself vocally when I joined the Cabinteely Gospel Choir. In those days, we still went to Mass every Sunday and I would sit there counting the lights or just mentally giving each of the parishioners a makeover in my head. But when the choir was formed it brought a whole new sense of entertainment to boring Mass and, having wanted to be in a gospel choir since I'd watched *Sister Act*, I signed myself up. Initially I sang just with the group, but I longed to sing a solo. I felt I had an inner gospel diva of Baptist Church proportions within me who was just dying to get out. Eventually I worked up the courage and put myself forward. I dreaded that it was going to be a repeat of my *West Side Story* school musical audition, but thankfully on the day my voice came out. At rehearsals I sang pop hit 'Shackles' by Mary Mary with my friend Rebekah, who had an incredible voice, and we got a massive round of applause from all the others in the choir. They were gobsmacked by our voices. That was it, Rebekah and I were snapping up all the hot solos from then on and rockin' them out on the altar every Sunday. You could see the people at Mass loved it. The earlier Masses were empty, but the 12:30 Mass, the one we sang at, was packed to the rafters. We could have charged an entrance fee. I absolutely loved the performance part of it and I campaigned for us to wear robes like a proper gospel choir. Mum and I even made a fab royal blue one on the sewing machine and I wore it down to rehearsals one night to show them a vision of their future, but the women in the choir, who were all older than me, were too scared to wear them. 'Ugh! This is so frustrating! Doesn't anyone else want to be a superstar like me? We need to take this to the next level, people! I'm talking swaying, dance routines, clapping, lights, headset microphones. We could be huge! There could be a world tour in this!' But my showbiz ideas weren't shared by everyone; most of them were just in it as a hobby. I won't lie, every Sunday I used to day-dream about a record executive approaching me after the service and offering me a record deal, but as I don't currently have any Grammy awards on my mantelpiece, that obviously never happened.

I remember receiving a phone call from Tony, the director of the gospel choir, telling me we'd been asked to sing at a televised Mass on RTÉ and asking if I would do a solo. 'You already know the answer to that, Tony! Yes! Of course I will!' This is gonna be on the telly! Woo hoo! I was thrilled. The first thing I did, and we have this on home video, is slather a green mud mask on my face and hop on the exercise bike I had just received as a Christmas present from Mum and Dad. While drinking a two-litre bottle of water, I laughingly told the camera, 'I have three days to lose three stone!'

*31 December 2001. Age: 22.*

You've taken a break from temp work. You left your receptionist job because you hated it so much. Wish you would find a nice job. Probably the biggest eye-opener for us as parents was to discover your amazing singing voice. I found it hard to hold back the tears the first time I sneaked down to the church to hear you sing. I say sneaked because you wouldn't let me go to see you. I was stunned. We are so proud of our children. I know I haven't written much in the past few years. The change in our lives has been so dramatic. Gavin and the new house have been the main reasons I haven't had very much spare time for writing but hopefully in 2002 I can start to write more and maybe your life will be more interesting to write about. I'll close off this year and book with these words. Julie-Ann you are the loveliest daughter anyone could ever ask for. Mike and I are delighted to call you our beloved daughter. Even if we don't say it very often we love you dearly and hope that life brings you all the lovely things you deserve. With all my love, Mum x.

This was the final entry in my Baby Book. I had given up on the idea of being a make-up artist at this point. I had done some jobs, but the fact that it was so insecure with one great high-paying job one minute and then nothing for weeks was very frustrating and disheartening. I decided my next career choice was to be a pop star. I was having my voice trained with a vocal coach, who incidentally also trained Bono (you know me, I don't do things by halves) and when Louis Walsh's *Pop Stars* auditions rolled into town in 2001, I was down like a hot snot. When I got to the Tara Towers hotel where the auditions were being held and saw all the other people, my confidence immediately receded. You know why? Because I was surrounded by girls in hot pants and belly-tops and I felt like a human monster truck beside them. I couldn't get my head straight as I was so conscious of my appearance because I was overweight and, yep, it was

*West Side Story* take two when I stood up there in front of Louis Walsh, trembling at a nine on the Richter scale. I sounded like a dead church mouse. After that I felt I was too fat to ever be a pop star, so I quashed that dream and stuck to singing in the gospel choir while still continually eating and dieting and hopelessly wondering what I was going to do with my life now.

### 3 April 2002. Age: 22.

Dear Jules & Barry,

This is our first time leaving our babies while we go on holiday. We are not sure if you are yet able to fend for yourselves and feel so guilty leaving you behind because you don't know how to do so many things. You can't cook yet, or iron, or wash clothes, or waken up by yourself, or know when you should go to bed, or budget money, or when to stop eating, we don't know how you will manage without us! And we don't know how we are going to react either if we come home to an untidy house! Barry, I have the tyres on my car set to explode if you try to take it for a ride. Remember, every time you hear the buzzer on the gate it could be Father Tom coming to give you his blessing. There is no point fighting either. I won't be there to take sides. I've spat in all the alcohol so don't even think about inviting your friends up for a drink. When you think of me think, 'What can I do to make Mum's life easier? I know – I'll clean the house and wash and iron all the clothes and if I get time I'll polish all the brass!' We hope to be home on Saturday the 11th early in the morning. But just in case we don't make it back – we want you to know how much we really love you. You're the best kids in the whole world. We couldn't have asked for better. We also want you to know how much money we have in the bank, €26,000,000, and when Uncle Gerry reads out our will you will find a codicil: 'If the house is spotless on the 11th it's all yours. If not, when Gerry inspects it, and you know what he's like – the money goes to the poor.' So, have a great time. Take every opportunity to enjoy yourselves in someone else's house. We'll bring you back some sweets. Get Mass. We'll be in touch. Take care of yourselves and the goldfish. Eat sensibly. Remember we love you so, so, so, so, so, so, so, so, so, so long as you're sensible and we love you so much too. Wish you were coming – to hold me upright!

All our love, Mum & Dad xxxxxxxx

P.S. I've left money for food in the fruit bowl.

This was probably the most fun I'd ever had in the supermarket. Barry and I rolled a trolley up and down the aisles like we were on an episode of *Supermarket Sweep* with Dale Winton. We bought everything that Mum would only buy on occasion. The shopping list included macaroni and cheese sauce, variety cereal packs, Raisin Splitz, Carte D'Or ice-cream, mini-pizzas and waffles, plenty of packets of crisps and multiple bars of chocolate. We also took full advantage of the free gaff and had some mates over for drinks. I tidied the place up afterwards so it was sparkling, yet Detective Mum still knew we'd had people over. 'We didn't. I'm telling you!' I laughed. 'You did. I know you did. And do you know how I know? Because there's a branch broken on my rhododendron outside and I know it was broken by a football and I know by the colour of the stem that it was done about three days ago.' The lads I had invited over had been playing football in the back garden. Mouth hanging open, I realised I had no defence and she'd just found me guilty as charged.

One day, this letter arrived out of the blue in the post.

*July 2002*

Hi Julie-Ann,

Just wanted to drop you a line to say hello since it has been ages (years more like) from

the time we last talked. It must be a minimum
of five years actually! Maybe you remember
me? Maybe you don't. It's Graham from the
Institute of Education. I wore that *Star Trek*
t-shirt to the first night social in Temple
Bar, the day we hung out in Stephen's Green
sunbathing with the girls. I was just hoping
to re-establish contact with you once again,
as I lost touch when I mislaid my old address
book, yet I found it in the attic. I am still
contactable at my old address in Donegal.
Drop me a line if you can. I hope you're well.
I'm still at university, Maynooth of all places
as I deferred my degree for a year.

Hope to hear from you, Graham.

*July 2002*

Dear Graham,

How's it going? I was very surprised to get
your letter yesterday! Talk about out of the
blue, but I'm glad you sent it. I rooted out my
old diary from 1997 for a full recap. Of course
I remember who you are! (How could you
forget, I'm sure you're thinking!) I remember
you and your floppy hair and *Star Trek* t-shirt
(hope to God you've binned that by now!)
My account of you in my diary is hysterical,
I even have the little notes you wrote to me

saying 'Can I walk you down to the bus stop?' taped onto the pages. We were so immature and nervous around each other, but looking back on it, it's really sweet. So where have those five years gone? Well I'm about to turn 23. I'm living at home with the parentals. For the last year I've been working in McCabes Wine Shop in Foxrock and I can genuinely say that I love my job. A lot of that has to do with my boss Damian as he has me in stitches laughing all day long. I walked into the shop and told him that all I know is that wine comes in a glass bottle and in two different colours, but I'm willing to learn and asked him if he'd give me a job? Which thankfully he did and he has become my sensei for all things vino and I have learned so much about the wonderful world of wine that now it's become a real passion. So what about you? Did you ever get into medicine after your years of trying and missing by five points? What are you doing in Maynooth? Are you there training to join the priesthood?! You have to write back and fill me in on all your adventures. So that's all for now. I haven't written this much since my exams!

Ciao, Jules (I use this name a lot now as I've grown out of Julie-Ann)

I never sent this letter to Graham and do you know why? Because I now weighed 14 stone and I thought that if we met up and he saw how much weight I'd put on in the five years since he'd last seen me, that he would projectile-vomit on the spot and say, 'You deceitful cow! How could you lure me here and then present me with this human wheelbarrow of lard when I was under the impression that I was going to see the slim, hot Jules I remember from school! You treacherous deceptor! Get out of my face before anyone sees me standing beside you and my reputation is ruined forever!'

This would be one of the many, many times my weight would dictate my decisions and hinder any chances I had of finding romance. The voice in my head had really begun tormenting me now about how my weight was spiralling out of control. I named the ominous voice of my inner bad bitch Siobhan, which is my name *as Gaeilge*. I gave her a name as she felt like a separate entity in my head. In my imagination, Siobhan looked like a very skinny, perfect version of me, wearing a black pencil skirt, white blouse, red pointy stilettos and secretary-type glasses. She was quite feline in appearance and her mane was always perfectly coiffed and her red lipstick eternally immaculate, probably because she never ate actual food.

Siobhan was the one who would tell me what I looked like when I looked in the mirror. Like something from *Mean Girls*, she'd say, 'Oh Jules, look at the amount of cellulite on the backs of your thighs. That is revolting. Can you imagine if any man ever saw that? He would be repulsed. Your arms are actually getting bigger by the minute, aren't they? No amount of fake tan is going to make them look better. Bingo wings and you're only in your early twenties! You do know it's long-sleeve tops for you from here on in, right? I mean, they're actually like tree trunks hanging off your shoulders. Do the world a favour and just start wearing more black and definitely start wearing more make-up. Obviously we can see your face is chubby, but you're a human, not a hamster, so you'd want to start contouring with bronzer to even try and mask the pillow face somewhat. By the way, I wouldn't even bother spending your money on waxing any more. I'm actually surprised they're not charging you extra to wax away the cobwebs. Men aren't coming near you. I mean, when was the last time a penis checked in to those lasagna lips anyway? So why would you even bother?'

Siobhan was a roarin' bitch. I couldn't get rid of her. She went with me everywhere. I wondered what I'd have to do to evict her, but I knew she'd just be like, 'Squatters rights, biatch. I ain't goin' nowhere!' Isn't it really fascinating how loud the thoughts in your head can be? I thought I was going mad when I started doing 'mini-bets'. What are they? Well, you know when you scrunch up a piece of paper and then say to yourself, 'If I throw this and get it into the bin, then today is going to be a great day' and you do and you miss, so you roll up another piece and keep shooting until you land it in? That. I did it all the time with all sorts of things. 'If I eat THIS banana, then today will be fantastic.' And pretty much told myself that if I dared to choose any of the other bananas from the bunch, then the rest of the day was doomed for failure. If I open a packet of tablets and it's the end of the box that has the leaflet sticking out, then that day is pretty much a write-off. Well, I'll think it for a few seconds and then forget about it. How ridiculous. Mad thing is, I still do it to this day. I told Barry about it at the time and he said, 'Oh yeah. Mini-bets. I do them all the time!' and I got a great sense of relief from that. I thought I had OCD and was losing my marbles. It is essentially gambling though, isn't it? I wonder is it a sign of an addictive personality?

God, this is really depresso with my life going to shite and my mind warping thanks to that crackpot Siobhan. So here are my favourite jokes I always tell taxi men when I'm pissed.

What do you call a sheep with no legs?

A cloud!

What do you call a spider with no legs?

A raisin!

What did the leper say to the prostitute?

Keep the tip!

Why did the pervert cross the road?

Because he couldn't get his knob out of the chicken!

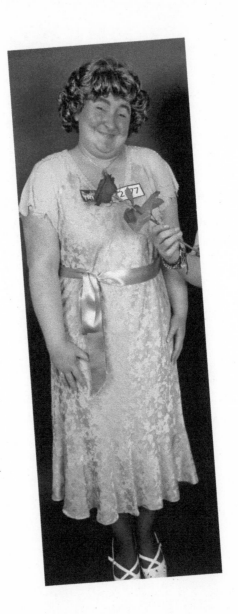

# 5

# Ovary Acting

*I* must admit to being rather pissed off that I didn't get a middle name when I was christened. As the years went by, I found it increasingly difficult to identify with the name Julie-Ann. It just didn't feel like me, so I adopted my nickname, Jules, on a full-time basis. Before this only my family and close friends called me Jules, so from my early twenties that's how I referred to myself with everyone, even for work where you're supposed to be formal. Feck that. Jules, that's me. That feels right. Julie-Ann is who I was when I made my Communion, but I ain't that little girl any more. I've just googled the meaning of my name and it tells me: 'Julie, meaning youthful, soft-haired, beautiful and vivacious' and Ann, meaning 'gracious, full of grace and mercy'. Well, Julie-Ann sounds like a right boring sap, doesn't she? Urban Dictionary tells me the meaning of the name Jules: 'The most amazing girlfriend anyone can ask for. Understanding, accepting, caring, loving, and hot as fuck.' Now that sounds more like it! But oh, the irony! I still can't get a boyfriend to save my life and yet that's the essence of the meaning of my name? Priceless. Maybe I should just go to the deed poll office and legally change my name to 'The One', actually that wouldn't work because everyone would just call me 'Yer Wan' for the laugh, wouldn't they? I think I'll just stick with Jules and be patient that I'll eventually become that 'amazing girlfriend'.

In my early twenties, when the Celtic Tiger was but a cub, myself and my cousin Renée strapped a saddle on his back and rode him like he was Battle Cat from *He-Man* and we were She-Ra and Sorceress. I was still doing shitty temp work, flitting from job to job and blowing all my income on socialising, while constantly trying to think of ingenious ways to become an instant millionaire. Money was flowing in the country again and we were right in the thick of the wad, living the high life with the beautiful people. We took a trip to Ladies' Day at Punchestown racecourse to swan around sipping Champagne and be 'lady-like'. Burberry's checkered print was totally on trend at the time, so after some heavy spending in Brown Thomas, I dressed myself from head to toe in their iconic print. I looked like a posh picnic. I had Burberry print boots, coat and matching bag and in order to complete my look I made a feather headpiece in the co-ordinating colours. With my giant Jackie O sunglasses, I secured a runner-up place in the Ladies' Day fashion competition and Renée bagged first prize with her fab lime green and pink ensemble. We knew we were on to a good thing when everyone was complimenting our feather creations. When our reply to 'Where did you buy them?' was 'We made them ourselves,' a business was born. We named it Eccentricks and we were convinced we were the next Phillip Treacy.

We set up a showroom from Renée's parents' house and ladies would come to us with their outfits for weddings or fancy events and we would dye feathers to match their threads and make custom feather fascinators to a style of their choice. Both very creative, as it turns out we were really good at it and every burn and blister from the lava hot glue gun was worth it as we were making a fortune. We initially made a name for Eccentricks by wearing the headpieces ourselves to events – the bigger, the better to attract more attention. I won a trip for two to the races in Cheltenham after I fixed a competition draw at a race meeting in Leopardstown by marking my ticket entry with a big red X, which was miraculously chosen from the barrel. When we flew over for the races, the lovely people in Aer Lingus even gave us our own seats for our extravagant bonnets. Mine was a large, black-rimmed hat that I had decorated with an erection of peacock feathers, while Renée wore a giant spider's web with a big beady-eyed spider resting on top of it. We loved the attention and posed for the paparazzi like we were Patsy and Eddie in *Ab Fab*. My pet peacock and I ended up on the front page of the *Irish Independent* the following day. We thought we were the flamingo's knickers. On the way home, in the airport a man in his seventies approached me and said, 'Oh I know you! You're the girl who was on the telly today at the races!' I spouted, 'Oh yah, you probably saw me on the big screen.' He replied, 'Yes! You're the girl with the limp!' No, not the girl with the gigantic peacock doing a mating dance on the top of her head, the girl with the limp. That is because I was wearing a pair of boots that were feckin' killing me. So I thought I looked like a sexy peacock, but in fact I looked like a lame duck.

Soon enough, all the beautiful people, socialites and models of Ireland were sprouting Eccentricks pieces from their heads and we had a press-book bursting at the seams with photos and articles from all the fancy magazines and newspapers. Business was booming for us as our feather headpieces were on sale in Brown Thomas, Selfridges in London and every chic boutique going. We got swept away by the social world and if there was an opening of an eyelid being celebrated, we were in attendance, hobnobbing with the yaw-yaw people and clinking glasses of bubbles while dishing out our business cards.

The Celtic Tiger's balls were the size of watermelons at this stage and money was flowing around Ireland like nobody's business. Life was so chi chi. I moved out of Mum and Dad's and in with Renée, to a sexy penthouse apartment in Ringsend near the city centre. This independence and having a few quid in my pocket gave me a new lease of life. Renée and I were both size 14/16, so there was great comfort in that as we could relate to each other so much, plus she is a gas legend and our wild ways, in every sense, made us the perfect partners in crime on every front. Our parties were legendary. For one of Renée's birthday celebrations, I forgot to order the birthday cake. So I rang the cake maker to explain my dilemma. I was told that 24 hours' notice was far too short to have a personalised cake made so, cheeky bitch that I was, thinking on the spot I replied, 'That's such a pity because the cake is in fact for actress Renée Zellweger who'll be in Dublin tomorrow night celebrating her birthday.' That, of course, changed everything and the following day I collected a spectacular *Bridget Jones*-themed cake that was so heavy it took two of us to lift it.

Of course, throughout all this time the pressure to look good was on. Both Renée and I were wearing each other's clothes and we were constantly dieting together. We were both in the same carriage on the yo-yo rollercoaster. On Monday we were on 'the diet', the one that was defo going to work this time. By the weekend we were off it and out on the lash, living it up in the VIP section of Annabelle's nightclub and getting absolutely steamboats. There's only one thing better than a glass of Champagne – a bottle! We were both as bad as each other and would always stop at Abrakebabra on the way home. So much so, we didn't even have to ask each other if we were going to be bold and get some sinful food. All we had to do was give each other 'the look', which was a sly smile and naughty eyes that indicated, 'Feck the diet, let's get cheese and garlic fries!' Then we'd order two lots each as one wasn't enough. 'Take us to the green neon palm trees please, mister taxi man!' It became a running joke. We were even able to place our order in Mandarin to the Chinese staff as we knew them all by name because we were such regular customers.

I remember a low point one morning, waking up with a gargantuan hangover and feeling so hungry that my tummy rumbles sounded like dubstep. We actually took the Abrakebabra bag from the night before out of the bin, microwaved what was left in it and ate it. We sat there in silence looking at each other with disdain and then said '*Nil desperandum!*' and discussed what new diet we'd start the following day. 'In the meantime, let's clear the fridge and presses of all the bad food so we're not tempted,' I'd say. 'Will we bin it all?' Renée would suggest. 'Jesus, no! We spent good money on those Sugar Puffs, they're like four quid a box! Let's eat all the shite now, to cure our hangovers, and just consider today to be a write-off. But tomorrow we will bring our A-game and own it with the new Low GI Ketone Slim Fat Fast Shakes we're getting in the chemist tomorrow morning! I've got a good feeling about them. They'll have us looking better than Victoria's Secret models in no time!' I'd assure her.

'Yeah! Deadly! Let's make toasted sambos to get rid of all that bread.'

'Great idea! Throw us over the block of cheese there. Nice one! We'll have this fridge wiped out in no time. We are such great kitchen cleaners, aren't we? We will be amazing wives someday, won't we?'

'Totally!'

You name a diet, I've been on it.

171

**Weight Watchers:** This was one of those ones where, like most of them, I lost 20 pounds and then put back on 30. It wrecked my head living life looking at everything through a filter of points and trying to calculate my daily intake throughout the day. And write down everything you've eaten in a log? Ain't nobody got time for that!

**Cayenne pepper and lemon juice:** This is the shortest diet I've been on. I hate spicy things, so I only lasted one sip.

**Herbalife:** Some rank-tasting shakes that you use as a food substitute. You blitzed them with fruit and yogurt. I look back on it now and realise it didn't work as I was just pumping sugar into myself.

**The British Heart Foundation diet:** I went on this purely because hot dogs were one of the things on the menu. Did it for a week and got sick of eating hot dogs.

**The cabbage soup diet:** I'd like to formally apologise for the damage to the ozone layer that I created while on this diet.

**Fat burner tablets:** I bought these in a body-building shop after being told to go in and do 'the secret wink' to the person working there and then they'd whip them out for you from under the counter. They were essentially high doses of caffeine that were designed to help you peak in the gym. I was taking them while lying on the sofa watching TV and having palpitations.

**Xenical tablets:** These were on prescription from the doctor. They prevented fat from your food being absorbed by your colon. Renée and I promised our doctor we'd embark on a very low-fat diet. Of course we didn't and continued eating McDonald's burgers and chips, only to get a rude awakening and see that the toilet bowl was covered in a slick of orange grease any time we went to the bathroom. I expected Greenpeace to arrive at the door any minute. This stuff also gave us the runs and we lived in perpetual fear of doing a fart as we'd end up with orange knickers that would have to be immediately binned.

**The juice cleanse diet:** The only thing this cleansed me of was my will to live.

**Chinese slimming tea:** This brew smelled exactly like an ashtray and essentially was just a laxative that gave you the green apple splatters and left you with an arse like a burst tomato. I've since heard that these 'skinny teas' are referred to as 'pregnancy teas' because so many girls take them, get diarrhoea and their contraceptive pill is messed up so they wind up preggers.

**Motivation Clinic:** This was a clinic I went to where they dealt with you one-on-one. I ditched it once I realised it was costing me a fortune in consultations and I was just buying their bars, soups and shakes, which were all highly processed and made me feel like shite.

**Food intolerance test:** I had a blood test to see what food I was intolerant to, so I could avoid it and lose weight. Turns out it was only carrots. Typical.

**SlimFast:** Another one full of crappy meal-replacement shakes. Rumour had it they turned into tapeworms in your stomach and ate any other food you consumed. I wished the rumour was true and of course put it to the test, but no, it wasn't.

**The Alice in Wonderland diet:** I ate and drank everything I saw in the hope it might solve all my problems.

**MyFitnessPal:** This is an app that helps you track everything you've eaten in a day, but I found I couldn't accurately record my food intake until they included 'a shit tonne' as a unit of measurement.

**Atkins:** Give up carbs? Over my bread body. This was the worst experience out of all of them. The idea was to completely eliminate carbs, thus throwing my body into a state of ketosis where it would think it was in an apocalyptic state and go straight to the fat reserves to gobble them up like PacMan to survive. I was supposed to eat protein and little else. So I spent my days eating sausages and cheese and hawing at Renée while asking her, 'Does my breath smell like nail varnish remover yet?' because that would indicate my body had gone into ketotic hypoglycaemia and that I was getting skinny. Within days, I was as constipated as a drug mule, my skin was pasty and I looked like a white dog shit. Of course the remedy was a laxative, so I got some from the pharmacy. It was Fybogel, a drink with psyllium husks guaranteed to evacuate my poor stagnant bowels. However, the drink was orange-flavoured and hence contained sugar. Unaware that I was committing carbicide, I was knocking them back and thus counteracting my ketosis as I continued to shovel a full fry into my face three times a day thinking I was Princess Protein. After a tortuous few weeks I lost weight, but then literally had a day-dream about a piece of toast and looked down and saw that my body had re-mortgaged itself with a high percentage of interest.

The most common diet, the one I was always on, was the Monday diet. I would lie in bed on a Sunday evening looking back at old photos of myself on my laptop, wishing I could be as slim as I was back when I thought I was a hippo. 'I was only a baby hippo then,' I'd think to myself. 'Now I'm looking like a fully grown adult hippo.' Then I would tell myself, 'Right, that's it. Tomorrow morning you are getting up and going to the gym and you are going to eat nothing but healthy food and THIS TIME you are going to fucking stick with it! Do you hear me now, Siobhan? I am doing it this time and you're going to shut the fuck up and start encouraging me instead of trying to tempt me with bad foods, okay?!' And Siobhan would just sit there casually filing her nails and ignoring me while sipping on a mojito and I could tell she was nearly looking forward to encouraging me to rhubarb crumble. All of my Monday diets would start off great. I would consider myself to be knowledgeable about nutrition so I'd know what to eat that was healthy and I would feel so wholesome and in control sailing around the supermarket with my trolley buying chia seeds and spinach. I'd prepare my food and after the first few days, I'd feel so fantastic I'd step on the scales and part of me actually expected to suddenly be at my goal weight. Siobhan, my bête noir, would sidle in and try to whisper sabotaging words in my ear about how I should just give up and get back on the chocolate, but I'd immediately cut her off and ram a cucumber down her throat to prevent her from swaying me off my healthy path.

Come the weekend, things would go one way or another. Like two well-worn paths diverging in a wood, I travelled both. One side of the fork would be the wall that I would hit and think, 'I'm tired. I'll just have a little treat to perk me up.' Boom. Diet over. The other side would be that Friday feeling. I'd beam radiance and feel so full of *joie de vivre* that I'd think, 'My tummy is flatter. I can even notice a difference in my skin with all the water I've been drinking. I feel lighter. In fact, I'm glowing, can you actually see me gleaming? I feel GREAT! Let's go out!' Siobhan would tell me, 'This is the best idea you've ever had!' and off I'd go out on the rip and get absolutely transmogrified, eat my way out of the inevitable hangover and promise myself on Sunday evening that I'd start again afresh tomorrow. I always found excuses to divert the diet. 'Well, this weekend is so-and-so's birthday so I literally *have* to go out on the lash for that. Then there's the wedding and then this and then that.' There was always something. Yes, Jules, it's called life. Life got in the way. All of these occasions I saw as valid excuses and every Monday was a miserable groundhog day. There's a reason why 'die' is in 'diet'.

By my mid-twenties, I still hadn't managed to bag myself a boyfriend. Renée had gotten married to the love of her life and moved to Galway and I moved back home with Mum and Dad while I looked for a place of my own. Even though business was booming, we shut down Eccentricks on a whim because we were 'so over it' and changed our phone numbers to avoid the aftermath. My love life was still an arid desert. There had only been two guys who I'd been 'seeing' for a month or two, but neither constituted a real relationship. One guy just smoked hash all day and I hated it. In the end I asked him to choose between me and the marijuana and he didn't have to think for long before picking the weed over me and I walked out the door. The following day, he phoned me to tell me he was in hospital with a collapsed lung. Karma! The other guy was just a twat and not worth talking about. I longed for a boyfriend. Someone to care about me and someone to love. Mum sat me down one day and told me that rumours had been circulating that I might be gay and afraid to come out of the closet. I was speechless. Mum was lovely about it. 'Now it's absolutely fine if you are gay and if you're afraid to come out, don't be.' 'I'm not gay!' I immediately cut her off. I remember going on the defensive and stating categorically that I was straight but just hadn't met the right guy yet.

I cried for days over it. It's the most upset I've ever been in my whole life, but it wasn't about the fact that people were assuming I was gay; that's a logical conclusion people could come to, seeing as I'd never had a boyfriend. It was the fact that people were talking about me behind my back. Me and my vacant love life were a topic of conversation and this upset me greatly. I went into a panic to try and find a boyfriend to prove that I liked the D, but at this stage I was never getting chatted up. I don't blame men for it though. I don't think they looked at me on a night out and thought, 'Ugh. I'm not chatting her up because she's fat.' I think that because I thought so little of myself, thanks to my poor self-image due to my weight, I believed that I was so unattractive I wasn't worth chatting up. Because of this, men had no other option but to reflect that back to me. If I had believed that I was attractive and lovable, then men would have mirrored that back to me and I'd be getting chatted up all the time. But my self-worth was non-existent, and so was my sex life. They say a sneeze is equivalent to 10% of an orgasm so I always looked forward to having a cold or, better still, the flu. If I didn't have my battery-operated bunny from Ann Summers, I probably would have ended up in prison for numerous murderous crimes. I was keeping Duracell in business. Along with sending myself Valentine's cards (how pathetically sad), I gave up all hope that I'd find a boyfriend as no men were ever interested in me. I would picture myself at the age of 50, living in a remote cottage with 70 cats, talking gibberish to myself, with a hairy chin, living off tinned food. I feckin' hate cats.

There was only one way that I found I could attract men and that was online, where I could hide my fat rolls behind the keyboard. I had profiles on dating websites and MySpace. My profile picture was from back when I was slim and I would type away full of confidence, letting my personality shine as the unsuspecting guy would think he was chatting to a slim, bubbly girl. I never met any of the guys in real life though, as I knew they'd be disappointed to be greeted by a 15-stone version of what they thought was their hot online date. Oh my God, I've just realised I'm a catfish! Jaysus! Chatting to guys on the internet was one of my favourite pastimes. I had been at it since the web came to Ireland, from the time before profile photos when you couldn't even see who you were chatting to.

*6 October 1998. Age: 19.*

You have been busy communicating with 'Lost' on the internet. Oh those days spent chatting. One weekend you had a 9-hour chat with him. Eventually you had to meet. You had never seen a picture of each other and you were severely disappointed, he was bald and like a stick insect and he thought you were a babe. Your nickname was Bond Girl so we now know that physical attraction is very important. The internet is really catching on, in the past three months it has grown from three million users to 30 million. Our computer is so slow. 75 pentium 1.2 meg hard drive.

When I was 19, I had the balls to meet that guy because back then I looked good. Now, in my late twenties, and having stacked on the pounds, I was more or less using the chats as an ego boost. I suppose I was actually trying to reassure myself that I still had my mojo and that if I was slim, then men would find me attractive as lots of them wanted to meet me in real life. I always came up with excuses as to why we couldn't meet face to face. I wonder if I lined up those guys I chatted to and showed them what I really looked like then, how many of them would say, 'I'd still date you because I know what your personality is like and that's what I'm attracted to most'? Well, I guess I'll never know.

The more weight I piled on, the more my hormones went berserk and the more irregular my periods became. I worried, even though I hadn't met my Mr Right, about what would happen when I did and we wanted to start a family. We'd have to be having sex 365 nights a year in the hope that one of those rides would get me pregnant. Now while that plan of nympho sex with my lucky future husband sounded fantastic, I knew that there was definitely something up with my menstrual cycle as I was now getting only one or two periods a year and they only lasted a day or two. The average woman goes through 9,120 tampons in a lifetime, but my mouse in the house was so rare, I was only buying one box of lady cigars a year. So I decided to pay a visit to my GP to see what he thought. I love my doctor because he's compassionate and genuinely cares. He doesn't just throw a prescription at me and tell me I'm grand. He's been our family GP since we were kids and has seen us through all sorts of ailments, including the time when Barry got a She-Ra figurine for his fourth birthday and peeled the holographic sticker off her crown, rolled it up into a little ball and put it up his nose, as you do, and then couldn't get it back down. Poor Dr Cosgrave had to be called over and take it out with a tweezers while Barry screamed blue murder. Anyway, I relayed my predicament about my absence of shark week to him and he suspected that I had a hormonal imbalance, so he did a blood test and sent me for an ultrasound to have a look at my ovaries.

I went to the Blackrock Clinic and sat in the waiting room after drinking two litres of water to fill my bladder so they could get a proper look inside my womb. With my legs crossed tightly, I prayed I wouldn't pee all over the hospital floor. Finally I was called in and they squirted some freezing cold gel onto my tummy and did an ultrasound. The cysts on my ovaries were immediately visible. Along with the results of my blood test, it led to a diagnosis of PCOS. P C O what? Polycystic Ovarian Syndrome. 'What the hell is that?' I enquired. 'Will I live?' I was told that it's very common and affects 20% of Irish women. Basically the ovaries malfunction and this leads to hormonal imbalances and a potential myriad of other symptoms, such as irregular periods or heavy periods, acne or excess hair growth. I was also told that PCOS makes you prone to weight gain. 'I'm sorry, baking powder? Makes me prone to weight gain?! So *that's* why I'm fat?! Because of my hormones?!' Well, I jumped off the hospital bed and skipped out the door. I would have clicked my heels together but I was too fat to jump that high. FINALLY an excuse for why I was overweight. It was my hormones. The whole time they have been at fault and they're the reason I'm piling on the pounds. I couldn't wait to tell everyone.

'Did ya hear Jules has the PCOS?'

'What's that when it's at home?'

'It means her hormones are all over the shop and that's why she is the size she is.'

'Are ya serious, Dymphna? The poor creature. Hormones can be a right bastard, so they can.'

'I hope she sorts them out and gets herself back slim again. She has such a lovely face. It's only desperate to see it lost in all the bloat, isn't it?'

'It is, Fidelma. It is.'

I wondered if I was part-panda. Sure they're living proof that you can just eat greens and still be fat. I was so happy that I'd found an excuse for being overweight that I hadn't even thought past what exactly PCOS was and what I could do about it. So I took to the internet to read up about it. Whenever I learn about anything medical, I always picture it in terms of the 1980s cartoon *How The Body Works*, which used to show us bodily functions with animated characters personifying all the systems in the body, like little men holding scrolls who would run at high speed through the nervous system delivering messages to the brain. So when it came to understanding PCOS, this is how I pictured it. In a normal menstrual cycle the ovary releases an egg once a month. This egg is pre-programmed to be a slut and is absolutely gagging to be impregnated. Wearing racy lingerie, she slides down the fallopian tube and lands in the uterus. This I picture as the dancefloor of Copper Face Jacks nightclub. Here she spritzes perfume on herself, applies red lipstick, lies on the bar seductively and says, 'Paint me like one of your French girls' as she waits for sperm to arrive and seduce her. When no jizz arrives, she knocks back a few tequilas and in a rage she begins to violently trash the place. This is period pain. Taking painkillers is like sending in a load of bouncers to restrain her. Exhausted, she then passes out on the red velvet sofas and workmen arrive to remove the furniture and she slips away into the abyss. This is the period itself.

In my reproductive system, things work a little differently. Up in the ovary, the eggs are all sleeping peacefully. Hormones arrive and wake one egg and tell her that she is 'The Chosen One' and present her with a Copper Face Jacks gold card entitling her to free entry into the club. Rather than sliding down the fallopian tube to get into the nightclub like she's supposed to, my ditzy egg cracks open a bottle of vodka and begins pre-drinking. She is a total lightweight and gets absolutely scuthered. Too blind drunk to even see the fallopian slide, she instead runs head-first into the wall of the ovary, bursts through it, knocks herself out and becomes a cyst. Meanwhile, tumbleweeds blow across the dance floor that is my uterus and I don't get any periods. I imagine that the DJ is a cricket sitting there rubbing his legs together, making cricket noises.

I took a trip back to see Dr Cosgrave and tell him of my diagnosis. At this stage I had begun to worry whether I'd ever be able to conceive. I figured that it was best to tackle my PCOS now, even though I didn't have a man in my life to procreate with, and then it'd be sorted when the time came to bake a bun in the oven. The first option was to go on the pill to regulate my periods. I hadn't been on it before as I'd had no need for contraception. 'This'll be grand,' I thought. 'You just pop a pill every day for three weeks and then you get a period. Easy.' A week on the poxy pill and I started to feel weird. I was an emotional wreck, bawling crying for absolutely no reason, and my usual cheery self had been replaced with a Jules that felt like I was having a constant out-of-body experience. It was like I wasn't even in my own carcass but outside of it, looking down on myself, like I was ghost. It's difficult to explain, but basically I just felt completely kooky and I longed to go back to feeling 'normal'. I endured it for a few months, but then chucked the pill in the bin once I'd realised the regular periods weren't worth the weirdness.

Back to the doc and he suggested I go to see a gynaecologist to investigate other options to sort my PCOS. So I did, but the one I picked turned out to be a right mega-bitch. She sat across from me at her desk and told me that the most effective solution for curing PCOS was to lose weight as that would regulate my hormones and give me regular periods. I told her, 'But I've been trying that for years, the PCOS makes me prone to putting on weight.' She put her elbows on her desk, folded her arms and said through a deadpan stare, 'Just-go-on-a-diet.' I was dumbfounded by her abruptness and in silence I paid her €250 fee for my five-minute consultation and walked out of her office. It was one of those situations when you're so shocked in the moment that you can't think of anything to say and it's not until you're walking back to your car that you think to yourself, why didn't I respond to her and say, 'Listen, biatch. I'm 27. I've been on a diet for eight years now! Eight feckin' years! I've tried them all and none of them work! I've tried to lose weight and I'm just getting bigger! Why don't you ... why don't you put your ugly face ... on a diet! You stupid ... stupid ... cow!' Instead of going back into her office and saying that, I drove to McDonald's and ordered half the menu.

Giving up on any hope of curing my PCOS, I decided to continue my perpetual dieting in the hope that one day I'd find a diet that worked and in the meantime I'd live without periods. It's funny how most women moan about having PMT, period pain and the bane of being up on blocks for a week every month. Whenever I got one, I'd text Mum to tell her because it was headline news. As my weight continued to spiral out of control, my self-loathing increased. I began eating more and more. I would whisper to my snacks, 'Let's take this upstairs,' then sit in bed eating toast, biscuits and chocolate bars. I felt that if nobody saw me eating the food, then it didn't count.

My secret eating was also done a lot in the car. I couldn't pull into the garage to get petrol without treating myself to a sandwich, a bag of Tayto crisps and a Moro. I drove more safely when there was food in my passenger seat than when there was a person sitting there. I began to notice that I was doing a lot of unconscious eating too. I'd stop at the traffic lights and look down at my lap and wonder where my KitKat had disappeared to. I didn't even remember eating it as I was on autopilot, shoving it into my mouth, obviously not even savouring the taste and just munching away as I drove along. When I realised I couldn't even remember eating things, I felt like someone had stolen the food right from under my nose. Sometimes I'd even check down the side of the seat to see if it had fallen, but no, there was never anything there. I had full-on food amnesia. The worst was the Maltesers. I'd put my hand in the bag and there'd only be one left. 'Where have the other 20 gone to?! Was this a dud bag?' I'd wonder. Faced with only one remaining Malteser, I'd put it in my mouth and try to make it last for as long as possible.

As my face dilated I found myself shying away from cameras when photos were being taken. I loved bringing my camera on a night out and would take pictures of everyone else, except myself. And if I did have to be in a photo, I would edit it afterwards and crop my body out of the shot and as long as it was taken at the right angle so my face didn't look too gigantic, I'd post it online, but most photos went into the virtual trash can. Therefore they didn't exist as far as I was concerned. I would dread seeing a notification on Facebook saying, 'You have been tagged in eight of Claire's photos' and I would quickly go and un-tag myself. Often I would have to message friends and ask them to remove particular pics as I couldn't bear the thought of them being online for all to see. When taking a selfie, I'd hold my phone up high so as to have the least amount of double chin possible. At one stage I was only short of hiring a crane to take the shot.

As if I was in mourning for my old slim body, I dressed in black from head to toe every day. My 'uniform' was black trousers made from soft, stretchy fabric with an elasticated waistband and a black top that had three-quarter length sleeves, elasticated under the bust line with flowy material that went to mid-thigh. This outfit was comfy, covered a multitude and blotted out my body so that I could promote the best thing I had going for me, which was, even though it was engulfed in fat, my face and my hair. I always made an effort with my make-up and hair, to show that I wasn't a lazy lump who'd just let herself go. No, I was a woman whose hormones were out to get her. I was a victim of my own endocrine system.

I only wore flat shoes as my size was so great at this stage that any form of a heel would bring so much weight to bear on the ball of my foot that it would feel like I'd been walking on hot coals. I cut the size labels off everything I bought as seeing size 18 tags would make me feel miserable. It was like, if they weren't there, then my clothes were just me size, whatever that was. So I wore my black uniform like Homer Simpson wears his, day in and day out, showing only my forearms and head. Everything else was covered in baggy black fabric. When I was going out I had a night-time version of my uniform, which had a few sequins around the neckline. I would look at all the fashionable clothes in the shops and wonder what it would be like to wear them. I constantly dreamed of the day I would be able to. When I saw a gorgeous coral-coloured tracksuit in a shop one day, I bought it in a size 14 and told myself I'd get into it. Little did I know it would sit unworn in my wardrobe for ten years.

Hanging alongside the coveted coral tracksuit in my wardrobe was an array of costumes. For most people, Hallowe'en means bonfires, trick-or-treating and fancy-dress costumes that you buy in a packet. For me, it's the ultimate creative day of the year. I plan my costume months in advance and over the years I've become renowned for the effort I put in. I just love the opportunity to become someone or something else. I suppose it's because it's a chance to escape being me and becoming a different character enables me to do that, if just for one night. My make-up training enabled me to turn myself into pretty much anything, well anything except skinny (I'm not that good!). I've dressed up as all sorts of personas and I always go all out with the endeavour.

It started from an early age in a school summer camp. I glued empty soft drinks cans all over a pair of tracksuit bottoms, stapled shredded newspaper to my sweatshirt and in case anyone wasn't aware (everyone) I hung a sign around my neck that read 'I Am Recycled'. Obviously, I looked like a right environmentalist, with the emphasis on the mentalist. Luckily my skills improved as the years went on. I've been a zombie bride in a blood-drenched gown. I've been Mother Teresa – the white sheet was very flattering to hide the flab, but I was pissed when I did the ageing make-up and ended up looking like E.T. when he's wrapped in the blanket sitting in the basket on the front of the bike at the end of the movie. I was 1980s Bridal Barbie in a puff-ball wedding dress, a school nerd complete with a minefield of pus-filled spots, bucked teeth and a 'KICK ME!' sign on my back … the list goes on.

One of my most embarrassing moments happened in fancy dress. Even though I'm a girl, I was so obsessed with Sasha Baron Cohen's comedy character Ali G that I dressed up as him. I shelled out 80 quid for the Fubu oversized yellow hoody, dyed a pair of white tracksuit bottoms yellow, stuck on the black goatee and donned his trademark yellow-tinted glasses and red Tommy Gear skull-cap. You could still see I had knockers under the tracksuit, so I referred to myself as Sally G for the night. I went out on the lash, saying

'Booyakasha! Easy now!' to everyone I met. Then I bumped into a guy who was also dressed as Ali G. He looked epic as his tracksuit was made from yellow PVC. The bastard. Where did he source that? In the club I was at they cleared the dance floor and the MC came out to announce the winners of the fancy-dress competition. He bellowed down the mic, 'And in third place, it's Ali G!' Pissed as a fart and absolutely delighted with myself, I breakdanced the robot out onto the dance floor to collect my prize only to be told, 'Sorry, love, not you, the other Ali G.' I'm going scarlet now just thinking about it. I had to sheepishly walk off back into the crowd as everyone looked on, no doubt saying, 'Oh my God, morto for your woman! What a dope!' Cringe.

In 2008, I was mad into watching *Little Britain* and I knew I just had to dress up as Vicky Pollard as I wanted to march around all night in costume saying, 'Yeah but no but yeah but no but' while swilling pints of cider. Vicky was fatter than me, so I had to stuff a pillow down the front of the pink Kappa tracksuit top. This made me feel great. At least my belly wasn't big enough to warrant fitting fully into character. I purchased a lovely long blonde wig and hacked it up with the scissors and then sprayed it with fake tan to make it look similar to Vicky's bad hair-dye job. I went out that Hallowe'en proudly pushing a buggy containing a big doll as my 'child', which I had dressed as a miniature version of my Vicky Pollard self. Vindication at last: I won first prize, which was €1,000. So of course, the subsequent year the pressure was on to out-do myself.

The following April one of the greatest television moments of all time aired when Scottish spinster Susan Boyle trundled on stage and auditioned for *Britain's Got Talent*. She took us all by storm with her eccentric banter and, of course, her incredible singing voice. She fascinated me. Her appearance was so idiosyncratic, she was a ready-made character. As the series progressed, I saw Susan's fame increase as the entire world looked on and warmed to her charms. Her initial audition on YouTube went viral like a coldsore at a teenage disco and everyone knew who she was. Bingo! I knew who I was dressing up as for Hallowe'en: the Hairy Angel.

Come October, I watched Susan's still popular audition on YouTube over and over, pausing repeatedly to study exactly what she was wearing. It's all about the details, you see. I wondered where in the name of 1980s curtains I was going to find a dress that resembled hers. If the worst came to the worst, I'd find some vintage drapes and make it from scratch, but that seemed like such a trek. So I headed into town to trawl the second-hand shops in the hope of striking it lucky and getting the perfect dress for a serious bargain. I have a remarkable ability to switch on what I call my 'costume blinkers' when I'm on the hunt shopping for something in particular. I'm like a pig sniffing out truffles and nothing can distract me from my mission.

First stop, charity shops. I stand outside and take a few deep breaths, knowing that I'm only going to be shallow breathing through my scarf once I enter. Why do these fusty second-hand bazaars always smell like dead people? Not that I even know what a dead person smells like, but the whiff in most of them can only be described as Eau de Morgue. I scramble rapidly through the racks, searching only for pale gold, frumpy dresses, but there's nothing but drab blouses and raincoats that have endured plenty of storms. It's the same result in the several other charity shops I bravely enter. Ah sure, it was a long shot anyway. After rifling through the final donation boutique I make a swift exit, gasping for breath. I give up. My plan to create the costume for under 20 quid has failed, so it's time to hit the real shops and go all out. At this stage I have envisioned the outcome in my head for so long I am determined to be SuBo, so I don't care if I'm going to shell out a few quid to make it happen.

I stroll excitedly through the doors of Arnotts and seek out the Grannies Department. I'm not sure if it's officially called that, but it's the section that has the classic knitwear, twin sets and 'lovely frocks', as they'd say down the bingo, ya know? I circulate around the racks, looking at all the pleated skirts in every shade of pastel imaginable. Is there a rule when you get to a certain old lady age that you're only allowed to wear mainly beige on most days and then break out the pastels for special occasions? Is it to complement the grey hair? We used to always slag my nana because she was beige from head to toe, like a human Lady Finger biscuit. I suppose they choose it because it's subdued and sure, it's an aul classic colour, isn't it? Goes with everything. Especially beige on beige. Wait! Hold the phone, Fidelma! Pale gold, fleur de lis-type print at three o'clock. Jackpot! I sprint over to what looks like a replica of SuBo's gold dress. Except it's a skirt and top. No problemo, I'll lash it through the sewing machine and stitch it together. I'll make a gold ribbon belt that will hide the join and it'll be perfect. I grab the size 16 and the size 18 and head to the fitting rooms.

Thankfully, the bias cut is very generous and the size 16 fits me perfectly. They must give grannies a bit of allowance for giant knockers and hips. Nice one. I tuck the top into the skirt, tilt my head to the side and squint as I look in the mirror to try and imagine what it will look like with the alterations. I can defo make this work. I smile smugly at my reflection and then place my fists on my hips and do the SuBo hip jiggle. It's going to be epic going out like this. The skirt length is mid-calf and I stand looking at my 'cankles' in the reflection. They look like my old school principal's legs. We used to call her Tree Trunks. I stare disappointedly for a few more moments, then shake my head and think, 'So what! Thank God SuBo wore tights so that'll cover them up a bit. I am going to look hilarious when I put this whole look together.' I undress and get back into my normal clothes, the usual black uniform, what else? I swish back the dressing-room curtain and I am greeted by a lovely sales assistant.

'How did you get on? Were you alright for sizes? I'd say the colour was gorgeous on you. Is it for a special occasion?' Oh God. 'Yeah, I'm dressing up as a singing spinster, it's perfect!' Do not say that out loud. Just play along. 'Yes, I'm very happy with it. I'm going to take it, thanks,' I tell her. 'Lovely. I'll take you over to the till. So is it for a wedding?' she asks. 'A wedding? Yes actually, a wedding, my … eh, yeah my cousin is getting married, so I just thought this would be nice for the day that's in it.' 'Ah sure, I'd say the gold is lovely with your sallow skin and the fabric is beautiful. You'll be a picture!' Please take my 85 quid and let me go. 'Wait now, what am I doing, I forgot to wrap it up in tissue paper so it doesn't crease.' I contemplate commenting on the weather just to change the subject as I pray she doesn't ask me for any more details about the fictional wedding I'm attending because I hate lying, but in a case like this the lies of the white kind are easier for both of us. She hands me the Arnotts bag. 'Well now, I hope you have a lovely time at the wedding and I hope you get a great day for it.' 'Thanks a million. I'm sure we will.' She is so sweet. I feel awful. I grab the bag and practically ski down the escalator to escape.

Two weeks to Hallowe'en, so I vow to abstain from my usual weekly basting of fake tan and instead revert to my traditional Irish corned beef skin *à la* Susan. The postman delivers my grey curly wig, which I ordered online from a wig shop in Hollywood, and the theatrical-quality men's grey stick-on eyebrows that came from a special FX make-up shop in London. Thanks to my costume blinkers, I find the perfect cream court shoes in Penney's for six quid. Then it's just 10-denier black tights, a print-out of the *Britain's Got Talent* contestant number to stick to my chest, an old microphone I found in a drawer and I've got all my components ready. The last day of October arrives and after making up Barry to look like Edward Scissorhands, as promised, I clear the decks in my bathroom and get ready to begin my transformation. I have all my make-up kit out and as I look at my pale face in the mirror, I wonder how long it's going to take to morph into SuBo. Surprisingly, it doesn't take as long as I expected. Fifteen minutes, to be exact.

If it's this quick to mutate into the Hairy Angel, I contemplate the fact that this can mean only two things: one, I am uglier than I originally thought; or two, I am such a blank canvas that I am chameleonic, just like the best models should be. Or perhaps I am just a very talented make-up artist? Yes, that's it. I'll go with that thought.

Gurning away in the mirror I think to myself that this is the first time ever that my double chin has come in handy! In fact, it's not even big enough so I am pressing down my chin into my neck and shading in the crease with glee. A bit more unflattering shading around eyes, jowls and delicately on my upper lip for a hint of menopausal moustache and I can see the contours of SuBo staring back at me. My trusty stipple sponge dipped in a wine-tinted crème make-up helps to create the blowsier broken veins. Finally, with the assistance of spirit gum, a very sticky glue that's safe to use on the skin, I apply the fake eyebrows. They're a bit creepy when you look at them up close as they're made from human hairs individually knotted through a mesh of skin-coloured netting. Not human eyebrow hair, but human head hair trimmed down. Still, equally as gross I suppose. I wonder where the hair comes from? Imagine they had that on donor cards. That'd be gas. 'In case of sudden death, I pledge to donate my heart, lungs, kidneys and hair. Sell it to a wig-maker. I won't need it in the afterlife. It was a pain in the ass to straighten every day anyway. I'll rock the Sinead O'Connor look in heaven. Leave the money you get for my hair to my children to see them through college.'

The grey curly wig was a bit too neat so I backcombed it to make it a bit more in keeping with Susan's lack-of-conditioner frazzled look. I lay my costume out on the bed. There is nothing like folding your own knickers to remind you how big your arse has become. To delay the satisfaction, I placed the wig on my head without looking in the mirror. I couldn't wait to get the gold dress on. Only then would I look at my reflection to assess the completed look. On with the tights, doing the 'tights dance' that every girl does as she wriggles them up her legs to ensure they snugly reach her crotch to prevent her thighs from rubbing together. Or am I the only one who does that? Shite! I forgot to shave my legs. Wait, this is actually a good thing. I laugh and tell myself I am more method than Daniel Day-Lewis. Not a chance I'm scoring tonight anyway, so I'm rolling with the cactus legs. On with the clumpy cream brogues. Thankfully they only have a one-inch heel, but I still pray that I'll be able to survive the night in them without developing third-degree bunions. I slip the frumpy gold dress off the hanger and throw it over my head, being careful not to smudge my ruddy complexion. The dress is surprisingly comfy. I figure grannies have it all worked out, just like those girls who rock around during the day in their pyjamas – comfort is the way forward. I step in front of the mirror and there she is. Hello Susan Boyle, you ol' Scottish legend! I have outdone myself this Hallowe'en and I can't wait to see people's reactions.

I strut downstairs and burst into the kitchen shouting in my best Scottish accent, 'Helloouu! Am Susan Bye-all!' Mum, Dad, Barry and Gavin are in knots laughing. Several million photos later we head over to my cousin Andy's gaff to crack into the pre-drinking. Andy and I were always close because he's a mad party animal like me. Everyone is in full costume and they go bananas when they see me. They've heard me rabbiting on about my SuBo for weeks and yes, I have delivered. 'How the hell did you get the red veins on your face?!' I explain the wonders of the stipple sponge. 'Oh my God, and you did it on your arms too? Amazing!' I hadn't done it on my arms. That was just my canned spam skin that hadn't seen the rays of the sun for several years minus the usual fake tan that masked it. 'Yeah, I had to make up my arms to match my face,' I lied. We milled into the booze and took a shedload of photos on my digital camera to be duly uploaded on Facebook the following morning. Remember, this was pre-mobile phone photo days, so you couldn't just snap a pic, pop it online and get an instant reaction. So I would have to wait until tomorrow to hook the camera to my laptop, upload and enjoy the likes and comments, but at least that would be something to entertain me during my anticipated colossal hangover. Little did I know that an instant reaction was awaiting me sooner than I expected. Tanked up on vodkas that were yet to kick in, we piled into taxis to head to Club 92 in Leopardstown, which was always the place to go for Hallowe'en as everyone made huge efforts with their costumes.

The moment I step out of the taxi outside the nightclub someone spots me, points and shouts, 'Susan Boyle!' and with that I am mobbed. It takes me an hour just to clear through the queue of people outside the club who want to take a selfie with me and I am loving it. Once in the club it's the same. Several people tell me I should be working as an impersonator and the club should be paying me for this appearance. My lovely friends kindly bring me drinks because I can't make it to the bar. This is a way bigger reaction than I'd even imagined. I bag third prize in the fancy-dress competition and everyone tells me I've been robbed. I couldn't give a shite as I'm having such a fantastic time! I don't even care how fat I look in all the photos I'm posing for. In fact, the fatter the better! Tonight I'm not Jules, I'm SuBo.

The following day when I post up the photo album of the previous night's madness on Facebook, the comments from my friends are all the same: 'Jules, you could be a professional Susan Boyle impersonator! The likeness is mental.' So my hungover hands hit the keyboard and I begin to search the internet for lookalike agencies. Turns out there are none in Ireland but loads in the UK. I email my best pictures to the biggest one. They have an Angelina Jolie lookalike on their books who looks like a carbon copy of her. I always shoot for the top and if these guys are the best, then I'm aiming for them. Within the hour, I receive a reply email, saying, 'Thank you for sending your photos to us. Unfortunately we can't take you on as you're a male impersonating a female.' Sorry, what?! You think I'm a bloke? And that there's a willy swinging under that dress? Half-laughing and half-crushed I reply and tell them that I realise that Jules is a unisex name but I am, in fact, a woman and this is me dressed up as Susan Boyle for Hallowe'en. Please see photo attached of my 'normal' self. They apologise profusely while praising my transformation and agree to put me on their books.

Weeks pass and nothing comes of it until one day the agency calls and tells me that one of the biggest tabloid newspapers in the UK has seen my before and after photos and would like to interview me. Result! The journalist phones that day and she is über nice, talking to me like we've been friends for years. She tells me they're sending a photographer around to my house that afternoon to take pictures of me as

SuBo. This is so exciting! I chat away and tell her my story about how I'm a make-up artist and how much I love fancy dress and how I was mobbed on Hallowe'en night. All is going well until she starts quizzing me about my personal life. How much do I earn as a make-up artist? How much could I make as a SuBo impersonator? Do I have a boyfriend? Will I ruin my chances of men ever fancying me if I go full-time with this? Whoa horsey! I don't like where this is going. What sort of a picture are they painting of me? And not just me, Susan as well. I decide to tell her that I think this interview wasn't a good idea and I don't want to continue it. I hang up the phone and call the lookalike agency to tell them what happened. They are very nice about it and tell me I don't have to do anything I don't want to. Phew. This whole impersonator thing was a bad idea and I'm glad it never even started.

The following morning at 7 a.m. my cousin Andy calls me. Bleary-eyed, I answer the phone, thinking something must be wrong if he's phoning this early.

'Hiya Ted. Everything okay?' (We refer to each other as Ted all the time.)

'Teddy, you're in the paper! A big two-page spread! It's deadly!'

My eyes pop out of my head.

'What the hell?! I told them I wasn't doing the interview!'

'Well it looks like they ran it anyway! It's great! The headline says "Boyle impersonator to make £250 an hour".'

'*What?!* What else does it say?!'

'Teddy, I'm dyslexic, I'd be here until next Christmas trying to read it out to ya! Get down to the shops quick!'

I whip off the duvet, throw on my tracksuit, no make-up, couldn't care less if I bump into every single person I've ever snogged, and I speed down to the shops to grab a copy. I am horrified as I read it and see that in order to complete the article, they've made up loads of things I didn't say. The worst misquote is 'I don't have a boyfriend and I'm a little rotund but I hope someone will see the funny side of me being a Susan Boyle impersonator and love me no matter how I look.' Rotund? In what world would I ever refer to myself as rotund? What an abysmal adjective. I don't know why, but I always think of a barrel when I hear that word. Rotund. Ugh.

Well, there's only one thing for it, I think, back into the shop for a coffee, croissant and a large bar of chocolate to give myself some sort of compensation for the pain of being called, in my head, a fucking barrel. Before I have time to drown my sorrows in caffeine and sugar, my phone rings. It's the lookalike agency. I sigh and answer. 'Jules! Did you see the paper? It's fantastic!' she exclaims. 'I can't believe they ran the article. I think I sound like a right twat in it,' I reply. 'Well, what would you say if I told you that I've had the two biggest breakfast TV shows in Britain on the phone all morning and there is now a bidding war between them to secure you as a guest tomorrow?!' I am silent. She continues, 'Now, Jules, I know this is all quite overwhelming but everyone is loving your SuBo story and if we play our cards right, you could make some serious money out of this.' My eyes light up and my pupils morph into pound signs. *Cha ching!* 'Go on,' I reply. 'On the back of this newspaper article, we can do the TV breakfast show tomorrow and then do the magazines, more papers and appearances, the whole lot. It will be bonkers for a few months, but if you're up for it, I suggest you just throw yourself into it and make as much money as possible while you can.' I think about it for about a nanosecond and reply, 'I'll do it!' 'Great! Pack your bag. You'll be flying to London today. I'll call you back with details!'

I fly to London that afternoon and when I walk out of the arrivals hall, there is a man in a black suit holding a sign with my name on it. I've always wanted to experience that. I can't believe they've sent a chauffeur for not so little old me. He takes my case and drives me in a slick black Mercedes to a swanky hotel where I check in. I'm absolutely buzzing in anticipation of appearing on breakfast telly to millions of people. Ha! The craic! That evening a camera crew arrives to pick me up as they want to film me out in public as SuBo, to see people's reactions. They laugh their heads off when I step out of the lift and meet them in the hotel reception. We go to Leicester Square and even before the cameraman has had time to set up his camera I am being mobbed by people looking for photos with SuBo. The Asian tourists are going especially nuts. They film all of this and then take me to a bar to film me as I stroll through to see people's reactions. There's another riot of selfies and one drunkard even gets down on bended knee and proposes to me. I play it up for the cameras and pretend I'm embarrassed, like virginal SuBo would be. I'm doing my best Charlie Chaplin-type acting, trying to talk as little as possible because my Scottish accent is brutal.

When filming is done, I head back to my hotel to get some sleep as I'm up at 4 a.m. to go to the studio for the live interview. I rip off the clumpy shoes as soon as I get in to my hotel room. Even though my feet are as bruised as a whore's punani, I feel great. I think I'll order room service. Perusing the menu, I look up and glance in the mirror and my face drops in sheer horror. I move closer to the mirror to zoom in on my reflection. Oh my God. I've only got ONE eyebrow! Where the hell is the other one gone?! I begin desperately searching for it. Is it stuck to my dress? In my wig? On the bottom of my shoe? The floor? Where is it and when did it fall off?! I shine the torch light from my phone on the carpet as I crawl across it, frantically combing it with my fingers like a primary school mother looking for head-lice. But my hairy eyebrow is nowhere to be found. After what feels like hours of searching, I conclude that it's somewhere in Leicester Square, drifting around in the wind. Why didn't I bring spares and how am I going to go on telly in a few hours with only one eyebrow?! Deep breaths. Deep breaths. Okay. Okay. Breathe. What would MacGyver do? I peel off the one remaining eyebrow I still have and stare at it as my brain goes into emergency creative mode. Boom! I know what I'll do! I'll cover my eyebrow area in spirit gum and then trim some hair off my wig and mash it into the glue and that'll give me some unruly brows! Genius! I breathe a sigh of relief. God, I hope it works.

I'm up at the crack of sparrows and making myself up as Jules. They want to introduce me on the show beforehand as my normal self and get people to text in and try and guess which celebrity I impersonate. I never got to hear what people did text in. I've only just thought about that now. I wonder who they said. Someone told me in a nightclub once that I looked like Ricki Lake. I slapped him across the face. Anyway, I plough on the foundation, knowing that the TV studio lights are going to be harsh. Another chauffeur collects me from the hotel and whisks me to the TV studio. It's gigantic and as we stroll past the spectacular sets for *Dancing with the Stars*, I realise how at home I feel in this world of backstage bustle. From the make-up room, we go live and they film me smiling at the camera while the presenters tell the viewers that I'm a celebrity impersonator and ask if they can guess who I'm going to turn myself into. That done, I start cleansing my face of my nice, flattering make-up and start to turn into SuBo, desperately trying to do it as fast as possible in case they return to film a teaser update and manage to catch me bare-faced as the real me. That is the version of myself I don't want anyone to see. Made-up Jules or SuBo, grand. In-between raw? Forget it. My MacGyver plan for the eyebrows works out okay, but it's not a patch on the wondrous stick-on fake eyebrows. I decide the only way to deal with it is to tell the truth when I get out there as it is actually a funny story about how one of my eyebrows is now floating around London somewhere. Perhaps a pigeon has eaten it?

As I stand behind the screen wall ready to go live, I am awash with a cocktail of nerves and adrenaline. Only millions of people watching. No pressure. I take a few deep breaths and just tell myself to enjoy it. Wait, what if Susan Boyle herself is at home tucking into a haggis sambo and tuning in? What will she think of me? No time to ponder, the headset-wearing crew member signals to me to get ready to go live. I delicately touch my Plan B eyebrows to make sure they're still there. They feel like pubes on my forehead. The presenters introduce me and I waddle out and do the infamous SuBo hip wiggle and they love it. The interview goes really well and they laugh at my dilemma about my eyebrow that went walkies. I manage to answer all of their questions without inadvertently insulting SuBo, as I don't want anyone to think I'm slagging her off by dressing up as her. I love her because she's such a character in every sense. Afterwards, I check my phone and see that there has been a barrage of emails from the Irish press, all wanting to interview me. I reply and tell them that I'm contracted to several international magazines now for exclusives and unfortunately I can't talk to them. I am so celeb right now. I do another appearance on an afternoon TV show and then fly back home that evening. In the following weeks, I do loads of interviews over the phone with magazines across the world. I remember talking to one magazine in New Zealand and just thinking to myself, 'This is bonkers!'

After learning off SuBo's audition verbatim I did several live gigs around Dublin, miming everything she said and sang in that now legendary five minutes of TV history. The audience reaction at the gigs was always great as SuBo was insanely famous at this stage. Mind you, she'd had a makeover and looked great, but I was sticking with Traditional SuBo. I think people warmed to her initial audition so much, they delighted in feeling as if they were seeing it live. As much as I enjoyed the live performances, the press attention was really stressing me out. My phone never stopped buzzing and after three weeks I was completely burnt out. How ridiculous does that sound? I'm not even an actual famous person, I'm just pretending to be one and I'm feeling like I need to check in to the Priory to destress.

Yet another phone call from the lookalike agency comes in – they must have me on speed-dial at this stage. They tell me that two more offers are in. One to cut the ribbon at the opening of an electrolysis clinic in Scotland, hairy SuBo and all that, and the other to do a tour of my live performance in a hotel in Las Vegas. 'I'm not doing it,' I tell them. 'This is all getting way out of hand. This is my Hallowe'en costume and now we're talking about Vegas?!' I was absolutely wrecked and just tired of being someone else. I wanted to go back to being Jules again. I was sick of SuBo and no longer even cared how much money was involved.

That's how knackered and overwhelmed I was by the whole thing. The agency was very nice about it and gave me time to reconsider my decision, but even a week later I was adamant that my impersonator days were over. It was great while it lasted and I made a shit-load of dosh, but if that's what it's like pretending to be famous, I can't even imagine what it's like for a real celebrity. In order to prevent me being enticed back into the world of SuBo I threw out the wig and donated the dress to a charity shop. I like to think that some lovely size 16 granny snapped it up for a tenner and was delighted with herself. Sure it'd be lovely to wear to a wedding, wouldn't it?

My SuBo transformation threw me back into the world of make-up artistry and I landed a job working for comedy impressionist Mario Rosenstock of *Gift Grub* fame. He was going on his first tour around Ireland and my job was to make him up as the multitude of characters he impersonated. I made his costumes and sourced the wigs and I waited side-stage like one of the guys in the pit stop at the Grand Prix. When he ran off, I stripped and dressed him in seconds, transforming him into different personas. What a fun job, and what a fantastic person to work with. The man is a genius and we had a great working relationship as he gave me so much creative freedom and encouragement. I had such respect for his talent and enjoyed the job so much, I went out of my way with my efforts and he genuinely recognised this and praised me for it. This backing only served to inspire me to work even harder. I'd get phone calls saying, 'Jules, I'm going on *The Late Late Show* tomorrow night and I need to be Michael Flatley', and I'd be straight out to the shops, walking miles to hunt down the perfect attire. Or else it would be 'I know it's a few hours to show time, but I've scrapped the opening scene and I'm now going to do Michael D. Higgins dressed as Johnny Cash. Can you sort that?' I'd laugh and sprint around Temple Bar looking for cowboy boots, a tasselled leather coat, guitar and a cowboy hat. Some of the costumes and props were mad. At one point I remember thinking, 'If the cops pulled me over right now, how could I explain that in the boot of my car I currently have an altar boy costume, a fake gun, 20 feet of fisherman's rope, a black PVC catsuit and a gimp mask?'

Shortly after my 30th birthday in 2009, I finally managed to save enough money to fly the nest and moved out of Mum and Dad's house. I moved in with my best friend, Donna, who is also my cousin, to a tiny, now I mean *tiny*, cottage in Donnybrook. It was so small that when people visited we would all be touching knees as we sat in a circle on fold-out chairs in the living room, drinking tea. It was an absolute kip, but we loved it. We lived on a staple diet of chicken-flavoured Super Noodles and pizza and we were perpetually out on the piss. Domino's

Pizza sent us vouchers, aka hangover cures, through the letterbox every week and we were their best customers. I had given up on dieting at this stage and given up on men. I had reached a point of trying as best I could to just enjoy life and be happy. And I was happy, just not with my physical appearance. I hated myself, but I lived in a warped bubble of denial, telling myself that if your thighs touched it meant you were one step close to being a mermaid. I also convinced myself I'd eventually find a magical easy solution to sort myself out. Reverse anorexia, is that a thing? If it is, I had it. In the meantime I just decided to get on with it and have fun with my life.

And I managed to do this, until certain events would upset me, like when I went to the National Ploughing Championships and couldn't get a pair of wellies to fit me because my legs were so big. Not even the men's ones would go near my colossal calves. In the end I had to buy a pair and cut them around the ankle and claim, 'They're not as sweaty on my legs this way. Ankle wellies are way cooler in every sense.' (This year I got my first pair of Ugg boots because I was finally able to fit into them. I've worn them so much they've given me a feckin' bunion, which is something I didn't think you were legally allowed to get until you were technically an 'old lady'. Jaysus.) Then there was the time I went to the Aran Islands and the plane we flew in was microscopic and we all had to be weighed before we got on and they arranged the seating positions of the five other passengers around me as I was the heaviest. The only good thing about being fat was that I didn't have a thigh gap, so that meant I could never accidentally drop my phone down the toilet.

Going on holidays was the worst. I'd have the aeroplane seatbelt maxed out around my belly and be conscious that my hips were pouring into the seat of the person next to me, so I'd sit as rigid as a three-day-old corpse for the whole flight. I dreaded the sun as the heat would just make me sweatier than I already was. And of course I was covered head to toe in black material, so the sweat just poured down my back like the River Liffey into my arse crack. Not a hope I was getting into a bikini, obviously, not even in front of just my three best girlfriends. Nope. No chance anyone was seeing my snowman-white rolls of flab. Instead I said, 'I'm not a big fan of the sun. It's so bad for your skin, it ages you like a pear in a hot-press and you end up with a face like a ball-bag. I'm just going to sit under the umbrella here and read my book.'

And there I would stay in my black maxi-dress and shrug cardigan to hide my arms. I'd be sweating so much that my make-up would run down my face and I'd look like a Salvador Dali painting. I wore huge Jackie O-type sunglasses but my face was so big and bloated at this stage that I just looked like John Lennon. I'd be baking like a Christmas turkey and longing to jump into the pool to cool off, but instead I persisted through the perspiration as my best friends sunbathed and I silently prayed for the day I could have the freedom to sunbathe with them. My feet and hands would swell in the heat, so much so I'd have to put them in buckets of iced water as I was sure the skin was going to crack. It felt like I'd been stung by a thousand bees and was in anaFATlactic shock. Well, you should be in shock Jules, because you're in your late twenties, you're five foot seven and you weigh 16 stone. You are officially obese. Oh shit.

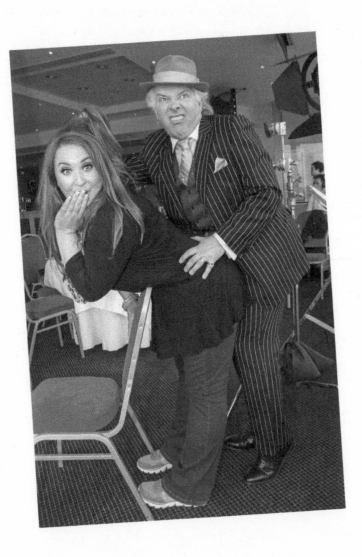

# 6

# Fatal Attraction

Would you be surprised if I told you that I have a side to me that's really into philosophy, spirituality, energy healing and all that lark? I am actually quite deep and poetic, I'll have you know. Here's a poem I wrote in school, aged 15.

*Me Spot*

I was lookin' in da mirror
and wha' did I see?
A huge red pussy pimple,
starin' back at me.

To da bathroom cabinet,
quickly I fled,
and out with da concealer
to hide me extra head.
I smeared it on, I rubbed it in,
But it did no good,
I should've known that bag o' chips
Would have me pullin' up me hood!
Ya couldn't see it from far back,
But when ya got up close,
Its shape 'n' colour made it look,
like a turkey roast.
I could see it when I crossed me eyes,
On da end o' me nose,
I mistook it for a strawberry whirl,
Eatin' me Cadbury's Rose.
To think of meself goin' out tonight,
Lookin' like a right fool,
I'll have to slap on a bandage
And just act really cool.

See? How deep and profound is that? Ah no, but seriously, I am very much into 'energy' and 'the universe' as I believe we are so much more than lemmings here on earth, plodding around like a pack of twats. There is so much more out there that we're unaware of.

I was raised a Catholic but by my late twenties I became disillusioned with the Catholic Church and its draconian ways and the threat of the Devil sticking his molten-lava pitchfork up my hole for all of eternity. I distanced myself from religion and instead found solace in alternative ways of being spiritual. Before this, when I thought of 'mind, body, spirit'-type people I thought of a tarot card-reading looper wearing a tie-dyed robe made from recycled plastic bottles and waving crystals and sage about the place. I didn't know anything about this world of energy healing until I experienced it for myself. It was Mum who delved into it first. She came back after a Reiki session raving about it, so much so I immediately booked myself in for an appointment.

I hadn't a rashers what to expect. When I got there, I thought I might be greeted by a hippie woman with mad, wiry, long grey hair wearing a long hemp-material skirt and a Rasta t-shirt with a peace symbol on the front of it who was going to read my palm and tell me I'd marry George Clooney, have seven children and become a billionaire all in the next 12 months. The person who met me at the door was quite the opposite. Her name was Kwan and she had long, dark hair, was of multiple mixed races and wore a white gown that was fit for a goddess. I sat opposite her and we talked about me and my life and then I started to 'see' the energy in the room. I know it sounds bonkers, but you know when you look at a lightbulb and then look away and you're left with that dazzling after-image in front of your eyes? Well, imagine that times a thousand all over the place. I also felt the energy and it was glorious. After our chat I lay on a massage table and she laid her hands on different parts of my body and I didn't know how it was happening, but I could feel an energetic resonance running through me that I'd never felt before. It felt divine, like I was being activated. We were so enthralled by this experience of feeling 'lighter', Mum and I began to study Reiki ourselves.

Reiki is a Japanese technique for stress relief and relaxation that also promotes healing. It's based on the idea that an invisible 'life-force energy' flows through us and is what gives us life. If our life-force energy is low, then we are more likely to get sick or feel stressed; if it is high, we are more capable of being happy and healthy. The word Reiki is made up of two Japanese words: *Rei*, which means 'The Higher Power'; and *Ki*, which means 'life-force energy'. So Reiki is actually 'spiritually guided life-force energy'.

Mum and I started studying it under the guidance of Kwan, our Reiki Master, and we found it so gratifying that it became a huge part of our lives. Over the course of several years, Mum and I trained to become Reiki Masters ourselves and we subsequently became Reiki practitioners and, as it turns out, we each have a particular gift for healing. I set up shop in a clinic in Rathmichael. It was such a rewarding job that it never felt like work. People would come to see me at the clinic and we'd chat about what they wanted to heal in their lives and then I would give them a Reiki treatment and clear everything we had discussed energetically and, kind of like a phone charger, I'd 'download' the Reiki energy through me and top up their energy battery. The results were astounding. I saw clients grow, heal and move forward in their lives. I can hear your asking, 'Well if they were all doing so great, why didn't you just Reiki yourself slim then, Jules?' I did. More about that later.

There were three incredible things I learned when I delved into the world of energy healing: the law of attraction; that all the world's a stage; and the mirrors philosophy.

So you've probably heard about the infamous book *The Secret* by Rhonda Byrne. When it first came out, there was huge worldwide hype surrounding it and everyone was raving about it. I was so intrigued to find out what this big secret was that, being the impatient wagon I am, I didn't even read the book but instead bought the DVD so I could get to the revelation as quickly as possible. It turns out that 'the secret' is the scientific law of attraction. *The Secret* posits that the law of attraction is a natural law that determines the complete order of the universe and of our personal lives through the process of 'like attracts like'. The author claims that as we think and feel, a corresponding frequency is sent out into the universe that attracts back to us events and circumstances on that same frequency. For example, if you think angry thoughts and feel angry, she claims that you will attract back events and circumstances that cause you to feel more anger. Conversely, if you think and feel positively, you will attract back positive events and circumstances. Proponents of the law claim that desirable outcomes, such as better health, wealth and happiness, can be attracted simply by changing one's thoughts and feelings. I started applying it to my life and it turns out it's a bang-on theory. To this day I live my life by it in every aspect.

All the world's a stage,
And all the men and women merely players;
They have their exits and their entrances;
And one man in his time plays many parts,
His acts being seven ages.

- William Shakespeare, *As You Like It*

Good ol' Shakey, he really knew his shit. The next principle I discovered is that all the world's a stage. Here is an analogy for how I imagine it: so I'm up in the lighting rig above a theatre stage that has big fancy red velvet curtains and all that jazz, and I'm the director and on stage are all the people in my life. Each of the 'actors', who are my family, friends, co-workers and randomers, are all holding scripts that I have written because they have all appeared, by the law of attraction, into my life to share experiences with me. Because I have written the scripts, each of them acts out their role to reflect back to me where I am in my life and what I need to experience. Each of them is, in fact, a mirror, which is what I mean by saying that I've written the script that they're acting out.

When I discovered the mirrors philosophy, it changed everything. I realised that everyone who came into my life was reflecting back what I was projecting and that this gave me an amazing opportunity to learn and heal myself. Here's a simple example of how it works: if I hold a belief that I am stupid, then I will attract into my life people and situations that make me feel stupid because this is what I believe about myself. I realised that they reflect my feelings of stupidity back to me so that I can see that belief in the mirror. So because of this, people whose personalities tended to upset or aggravate me became my greatest teachers.

This philosophy was initially difficult to comprehend. Take, for example, when Ciara (false name) came into my life. I couldn't stand her because she was so negative and critical about everyone. If someone was to come along and say to me, 'You know what, Jules, Ciara's not actually the problem here – you are,' what would the unhealed me have said? Probably, 'ya wha'?! Ciara's a total bitch! She's the one with the issues! She's so critical! All she does is criticise everyone and everything! She's unbelievable and it absolutely wrecks my head! She's the problem, not me! I can't stand the wagon! I hope she dies roarin'!' Then if they were to say to me, 'Well, Jules, if the problem lies truly with Ciara and not you, then why does being around her affect you so negatively?' What else could I reply to that but, 'Ehhh ... I dunno.' 'So, Jules, what Ciara is actually doing is mirroring back to you an aspect of yourself that you need to heal. She's playing a monster version of all the criticising that you are in fact doing to yourself and others.' The mirroring is often magnified to get our attention. 'Do you ever criticise anyone or anything, Jules?' My reply: 'Suppose.' 'What about yourself? Do you criticise yourself?' My answer: 'That's all I do. All the time. I look in the mirror and I criticise myself. Most of my thoughts are me chastising myself, if I'm honest.' 'So there we go. Ciara has to step onto your stage and play the role of Critical Ciara to mirror back to you the aspect of yourself that you need to heal.' It's so easy to point the finger and think that Ciara's the one with the issues, but I attracted her so she's here to teach me something.

So once I understood the mirrors idea, I started applying it to my life. As soon as someone upset or annoyed me, I'd take a deep breath and ask myself, 'What would I accuse them of?' And I'd name a list of words to describe my accusations. In the case of Ciara, I'd accuse her of being critical. Then I'd ask myself, 'When in my life am I critical?', and I'd look for the answer. And I'd know straightaway that I was being overly critical of myself and others. Then I'd acknowledge the realisation of what I needed to work on and then affirm, 'I now choose to release the aspect of myself that is overly critical. I will work on this for the next 21 days to create a new habit. Each time I find myself being critical I will be aware of it and instead will counteract it with a compliment to myself: 'Jules, you are feckin' great. You are a ride and you are beautiful inside and out.' Once I'd cleared and healed that aspect of myself, Ciara no longer needed to reflect it back to me, so she'd either step out of my life and tell me she was moving to Timbuktu or else she would suddenly stop being critical because her role in my life had now changed. I had rewritten her script. We miraculously ghosted each other and I never heard from her again. Jog on, Critical Ciara! Jog on! I realised that while blaming other people was very convenient, it's not always so easy. Once I'd grasped this, instead of avoiding these people and saying I didn't like them, I now knew that what I needed to do was to change my belief and then the reflection would change. I realised it was always about ME and not the other person. Always. I am the projector of it all.

Before realising this, what I usually tended to do when a person upset me was to avoid them in the hope that they wouldn't be around to wreck my head. I soon realised that it doesn't necessarily work that way. I suppose that's why some people tend to repeatedly attract partners with similar personal issues (cheaters, abusers, etc.). I saw that if I ran away from the person without learning the lesson from the relationship, then I'd very soon meet another person who would reflect the same image back to me. That would present a second opportunity for me to heal. If I didn't cop on then, it was on to a third and a fourth until I got the BIG picture landed in my lap and finally began the process of change and healing. I also realised that I serve as a mirror for others in my life without consciously realising it. That's why I find myself acting differently around different people, because I'm subconsciously acting out their script.

I apply the mirrors philosophy to myself all the time and it is always bang-on in reflecting back an aspect of myself that I need to work on. It's important to note too that all the people in my life who I've attracted onto my stage whom I love reflect back all the positive aspects of me. I found in my personal growth that it was so easy to just look at the negative stuff, but noting the positive mirror reflections is just as vital. I found that a great way of noticing how the mirrors work was to look at what celebrities attracted the press to write about them. 'Model seen looking dangerously thin at awards ceremony': now that could mean that this model believes that she is too thin or else she believes she's too big. Her core belief will attract that headline because that's what she needs to heal.

While I loved my job as a Reiki practitioner, after a few years doing it I realised that I was making everyone else's dreams come true and sorting everyone else's lives out, but what about my own? I needed to express myself creatively again and I knew that I desperately missed the world of TV and make-up artistry. So in 2009 I decided to just keep up the Reiki practice on myself and my own life and return to the world of telly and showbiz because I missed it and felt so at home there.

*Father Ted* is shite. There's a sentence you'll never hear. Isn't it great in Ireland that if you ever forget someone's name you can just call them Ted and it's universally accepted as every Irish person's nickname? Male or female, it works a charm. We've all done it. You're in the pub and you see so-and-so from back in the day and you can't for the life of you remember their name. You panic, running through the alphabet in your head: 'A… Alan, Andrew, Anthony, B… Bill, Barry, Bob… Shite, he's seen me. He's approaching. C… Colm, Caterpillar, Connor, D… Derek, Dildo … too late.' 'Jules! Long time no see! How are ya?!' And your face lights up full of sincerity as you say 'Ah howeya Ted! Are ya well?' And you slap each other on the back affectionately while thinking 'God bless *Father Ted*.' You chat away to Ted, only half listening to what he's saying as you're still mentally alphabetising while also thinking, 'he looks like a Niall. Maybe it's Niall? Or is it Neil?' and then suddenly the filing cabinet of your brain unlocks the correct file in your memory bank and you remember. 'Gareth! Yes! That's the one. Gareth from that party in Dave's gaff when we had that sing-song until six in the morning and I fed the dog guacamole and it puked everywhere!' So proud of yourself that you remembered his name, you then feel the urge to use it at every opportunity. 'So, Gareth, how's work?' 'Are you still playing the guitar, Gareth?' 'Oh Gareth, remember that sing-song we had and Jeff tried to hit the Celine Dion high note so he stood up and then fell through the coffee table?' 'Oh Gareth, that was gas, wasn't it? Great days, Gareth, great days.' 'Hey everyone, come and meet my mate Gareth!'

*Father Ted.* What a TV show. It'll never be topped and two decades on it's still funny and always will be. In my extended family for the past 20 years we've all been calling each other Ted or, for an even more affectionate attribute, Teddy. Our family coat-of-arms is a strait-jacket. Is that normal? We are a very close family. All of my cousins are my best mates and we have grown up spending a huge amount of time together. Andy, my madcap cousin, who's six years younger than me, is the acting talent of the family. He created the comedy characters Damo and Ivor. In the highly unlikely event that you don't know who Damo and Ivor are, they are a satirical comedy duo of cartoonish proportions and Andy, chameleon actor that he is, plays both parts. Their backstory is that they are identical twins, separated at birth and unaware of each other's existence. Damo grows up in a working-class life on the mean streets of inner-city Dublin, while Ivor's life is the opposite as he's from the posh world of affluence.

They both have trademark looks. Damo wears a red jacket, a big gold chain and a white cap with a 12-inch peak. Ivor's signature attire is beige chinos, brown Dubes and a pastel polo shirt with a six-inch erect collar, making him look somewhat like a dog wearing one of those cones the vet puts on him to stop him licking his balls. After using his mum's home video camera to make videos recreating Pat Shortt's sketches from *D'Unbelievables*, Andy decided to branch out and create his own comedy personas. First came Damo and his infamous *Skanger Me Banger* sketch, which was like a boy racer version of MTV's *Pimp My Ride*. It was the No. 1 video in the Bebo flashbox back in the day, with over one million views. This was before YouTube and before what we now know today as viral videos. Gangnam Style, feck right off.

As a family we are always very supportive of each other, especially when it comes to creativity. It was big news when, at the age of 16, Andy had his photo taken with Pat Shortt after watching him live at Vicar Street.

'Did you hear Andy met Pat Shortt?'

'I know! I saw the photo up on the fridge! Sure he'll be up on stage with him in no time!'

One day in early 2009 Andy showed me a copybook he had filled with drawings of Damo and Ivor in different scenarios. Being dyslexic, he struggled to write down the words that he was thinking so instead he drew them as cartoons. He talked me through some of the sketches and I was laughing my head off.

'Teddy, these are so funny! Do you want me to help you? I'm like lightning with the typing and you can just tell me what you want to write down and then you could have a script to shop around!'

'Are ya serious, Teddy?! That'd be amazing!'

He was thrilled. I told him, 'Now I haven't a rashers how to structure a film script, but we'll learn.' Thanks to a very helpful section on the BBC's Writer's Room website, I discovered how to format a script and off we started. Initially it started out with Andy dictating and me bashing away on the keyboard like a lunatic. It was great craic, and I was so inspired by the whole thing I started bouncing out ideas too. Before we knew it, we had become a writing duo. 'Feck the make-up artistry! I want to be a scriptwriter!' I thought. And even if that meant delving into my savings and living frugally so I could dedicate myself to it, then that's what I would do. Over the course of the summer our minds forged together and smelted an epic storyline and a load of gags for *Damo & Ivor*. We used to sit out in the gazebo with the laptop, chain-smoking like Colin Farrell after a long-haul flight, chugging coffee and laughing our heads off coming up with the funnies. We were rockin' it out, or so we thought. In July we broke open the Champagne and Waterford Crystal glasses to celebrate our finished script. It was about half an inch thick. We thought we'd written a movie. A proper script would be about two inches thick. What a pair of plonkers. Little did we know how long and arduous was the road that lay ahead.

We both loved what we were doing. TV is in our blood, you see. Both our mums, Jan and Ann, worked as film editors in Silverpine Studios in Bray, County Wicklow, which was set up by my late grandfather William Stapleton. In 1956, seven years before RTÉ even existed, my eccentric genius grandfather created Ireland's first television station and was the first person to produce and broadcast programmes on closed-circuit television in Ireland. I've had a thing for TV from an early age, always viewing shows and wondering what was going on behind the camera during each scene. And I'm obsessed with looking for continuity errors. I remember as a small child going into my grandfather's studio where they would develop the 16 and 35 mm film in gigantic machines. The intoxicating smell of the developing fluid was so distinctive. I would stand and watch the film reels racing through the troughs of chemicals. It probably made me high as a giraffe's balls. I loved it. Junkie Jules, age five.

We shopped our script around to a load of production companies and got lots of rejection letters. Never disheartened, we continued our uphill battle to reach an audience. We are ridiculously tenacious with our positive thinking. The one production company we had both dreamed of working with from the start was Parallel Films. Based in Dublin city, they've made legendary TV series and films, including black comedy *Intermission*, which Andy and I both adored. So I phoned them up one day and asked could we send in a script. I was politely told that they didn't accept scripts unless they came through an agent and not to send one as unsolicited scripts were, sadly, just put in the bin. I hung up the phone and said to Andy, 'Agent? Pah! Throw us a luminous yellow envelope there, will ya?' We sent off the script with a DVD of *Skanger Me Banger* and a load of photographs of Damo and Ivor. A picture paints a million words, as they say.

Miraculously, our eye-catching envelope landed on the desk of the right person, the amazing producer Ruth Carter. She later told us that when all the colourful photos slid out of the envelope, she knew she had to take a further look. Ruth watched the DVD and, thankfully, it made her laugh and she knew she was on to something. She phoned and arranged a meeting with us. Imagine that, rejected by every single one except the production company we most wanted to work with. That's providence in action. Providence meaning, 'A manifestation of divine care or direction', which is why when it came to choosing a name for the production company we later set up, we called it Providence Pictures. I knew at this stage that my healing work was graduating from working with individuals to working on a much bigger scale. My new path was to widely dispense the greatest medicine of all: laughter.

We met Ruth in March 2010 and she was keen on the project from the start. She told us that our scripts were all over the shop and that she thought *Damo & Ivor* would work better in the format of a TV show rather than a film, but that we had potential. We had found someone who believed in us. That's all the kick-start we needed. I remember at the time Ruth telling us that making a TV show was a long process and they had some people on their books for three or four years who were only now getting their projects to fruition. I couldn't believe that and I came out of the meeting going, 'Who are those saps hanging around for years trying to make a project materialise? Surely it can't take that long? They should just get a life and move on.' Little did I know! We went back to the drawing board and worked on the scripts intensely and came up with loads more material. The funny parts were easy for us, it was all the storyline bollocks and characters' motivation crap that we struggled with because we found it boring. We just wanted to write the funnies. But you can't put your make-up on without moisturising first.

While we were working, my diet was horrendous. We were writing intensely, sometimes up to 14 hours a day, so I was just fuelling myself with crap food to keep myself buzzing. I was drinking three cans of Red Bull per day. That's nearly 20 teaspoons of sugar and probably enough caffeine to reverse an anaesthetic.

And according to serving sizes, I was a family of four. I lived on baguette rolls filled with sausages, mayonnaise and ketchup, with a side of crisps, plus we had a ritual at 4 p.m. every day of driving down to the shop to get a Dairy Milk bar to have with a lovely cup of tea. Andy has the metabolism of a cheetah. He could pack away the food and stay slim. He didn't even work out and he was like Hercules. I was a human fat factory, expanding by the week.

A year later we were tired of looking at pieces of paper so we decided to bring *Damo & Ivor* to life. We wrote our first comedy song, called 'Everybody's Drinkin''. We enlisted two brilliant music producers and recorded the track and then got to work on the video. Now bear in mind, I'm a make-up artist, not a camerawoman, and we had little or no money, so how on earth were we going to do this? We pooled our savings and came up with two and half grand between us. To get a music video done with a production company was going to cost at least five times that, so we decided to do it ourselves on this little budget. I filmed and directed the video while Andy worked his magic in front of the camera. With a lot of hard work and help from all our friends coming in as extras, the finished product was epic.

Once the music video was edited we yet again set forth with high hopes and aimed for the top. I sent the video to *Republic of Telly* host Dermot Whelan. He was a friend on Twitter, but at the time I'd never met him in real life. Dermot loved it and showed it to James Cotter, the series producer in RTÉ. I'll always remember where we were when James phoned: Eason's bookshop in Dundrum. I took the call and mouthed to Andy, 'It's *Republic of Telly* on the phone!' Cue frantic hand flailing from me and a big 'What's he saying?' ecstatic face on Andy. James asked who we were and I told him. He then asked who the guys were playing Damo and Ivor. I told him it was one guy. James couldn't believe it. He told me he loved the video and wanted to show it on *Republic of Telly*. Woo hoo! We immediately legged it to Tesco, to the booze aisle, to buy cheap fizzy wine to spray in the air as we couldn't afford Champagne.

When the video aired on *Republic of Telly* on 18 April 2011, I was blown away by the way it happened. 'Everybody's Drinkin'' went live on YouTube immediately after it appeared on the show. We had no experience of watching something 'go viral' and it was just insane to watch. I didn't know that in ten seconds the view count would get stuck at 301 as there were so many views coming in at once, it would take YouTube up to 12 hours to process them and give a view count total. The song went to No. 1 on the iTunes music charts by seven o'clock the following morning. The press phone calls flooded in and on the advice of the fab Mario Rosenstock, Andy did all the interviews in character as Damo and Ivor and that worked really well. At that stage it was 50/50 between the fans as to who knew that both characters were played by one guy. Every day there'd be a comment war on YouTube between people:

'It IS the same guy!'

'It's not! They have different body shapes!'

'Yeah! Ivor has a butt chin!'

'It's TWO PEOPLE! Dey look nothin' like each other, ya fuckin' dope.'

In the music video we included a three-second video-clip of me dressed up as a skanger from Andy's 25th birthday party a year previously. I had my hair scraped back with wet-look hair gel into a high ponytail, aggressive eyeliner, a white Adidas tracksuit, which I'd had to purchase in the men's section of TK Maxx to get one big enough to fit me, a load of gold chains, tattoos of scorpions on me tits, a pair of white raver gloves and a black eye that I'd painted on with make-up. I looked so 100% skanger that we dropped the clip into the music video for the laugh. It led to loads of comments:

'Did ya see the head on your one at 1 minute 46?
Hahaha!'

'In bits laughin' at the cut of the skanger at 1:46.
Proper scummer! Deadly!'

I became known as 'the 1:46 bird'. I love being
a skanger. I called meself DJ Deirdre. When I'm
dressed up as her, I even walk differently. She is the
total opposite to my personality as she's so tetchy and
aggressive. One of those 'Wha' are you lookin' at?!
Are ya startin', are ya? Come near me and I'll burst ya!
D'ya hear me, ye tick?!' types.

I absolutely love playing an aggro character as I
never get to vent any anger like that in real life. I hate
confrontation and always avoid it. If anything, I'm
the opposite. Mum calls me 'The Buffer' because if I
even see any potential battles brewing between others,
I will slide in and, usually with humour, try to lighten
the situation to prevent any disputes detonating.
I don't know whether this is a positive or negative
attribute. Perhaps sometimes it's good to discharge
feelings and air grievances but I just don't like anyone,
myself included, to be in pain. I just want everyone
to be happy and in harmony. I couldn't explode on
someone like a volcano and blow lava in their face.
I just can't do it. Instead, I choose to go higher and
apply the mirrors philosophy and see what I need to

learn from the situation. Just call me Mrs Miyagi. Wax on. Wax off.

So now, fast forward through 2011. We continued to build the brand by making more successful viral comedy music videos, still producing them ourselves, and sketches for *Republic of Telly*, which was a great platform. I won't lie though, giving up production and editorial control on the TV sketches was really difficult. Especially for a perfectionist like me. We loved making the music videos the most as we had creative control over them. As we gained more experience, the creative ideas got bigger and bolder. The Christmas music video was my favourite – especially as I got to build a two-foot pyramid of Ferrero Rocher chocolates to feature in it. One for the pyramid. One for me. One for the pyramid. One for me. 'Andy, we're gonna need more chocolates!' We just knew we had to go to Lapland to shoot the video in a magical winter wonderland. It would have been rude not to. It was a total trek to get there as it was mid-November, so it was off-season. Three flights later and as we flew in to Rovaniemi, I looked out the window of the plane and then turned to Andy and said, 'There's no snow!' He laughed, 'Yeah, good one, Jules! We're at the actual North Pole, there has to be buckets of snow out there! The weather app says it's minus 19!' We landed. No snow. Could. Not. Believe. It.

Checked in at the Santa Claus Hotel and asked the receptionist, 'Are we being secretly filmed by *Punk'd?*' She just told me that it was global warming and there might be snow next week. We went straight to the bar and ordered double vodkas. We'd flown thousands of miles thinking we were going to a snowy oasis and there wasn't even a bit of dandruff floating around. So Operation 'What would MacGyver do?' was launched. Plan A was to go to a supermarket and buy a few thousand packets of icing sugar to sprinkle about the place. Plan B was to get in a taxi and trek three hours up the mountains to where there definitely was snow. We ploughed into the vodka and ordered a taxi for the following morning.

I fell asleep on the way there, practically drooling on the taxi man's shoulder, and woke up in a glistening whiteout. It was spectacular! We stopped and filmed some reindeer that were just frolicking on the side of the road, like a scene in a snow-globe. Then we passed some quaint log cabin-type houses and pulled in, legged it into their back garden and started filming Damo audaciously kicking the snow off the trees. Thank God the house owners weren't at home. If they had come out, our plan was to do a runner back to the car. When you're filming with Damo, you start thinking like him.

It was minus 25 degrees up in the mountains and the cold was indescribable. There are no runny noses in

Lapland because your snots are literally crystallised. We visited Santa's Village and we were thrilled when they gave us permission to film Damo with Santa Claus. He is definitely the real Santy. He was just so lovely, standing at six foot five with his glowing cheeks and his perfectly curly beard down to his knees. He can speak ten different languages. I think Santy was a bit baffled when he saw Damo coming in with the outlandish gold chain, a sovereign on every finger and the big peaked cap, but thankfully he went with it and we got some great shots. We hit the empty hotel bar that night in our pyjamas like a pair of skangers. There's defo something magical in the Finnish vodka because I didn't get any hangovers from it. The Russian stuff is shite.

The next day Andy shaved off his ronnie and transformed into Ivor and we flung ourselves into the taxi to repeat the same journey in search of snow. It had rained that night so the snow wasn't as powdery, but we found a good snowy bank at the entrance to a ski resort and filmed Ivor frolicking through the blizzard. Finally we visited Santa Park, where they had an ice bar. The Ice Queen gave us shots of cranberry vodka in shot glasses made of ice. We were skulling them back until I clocked the sign and realised they were 12 quid each. Twelve quid! I felt like vomiting it back into the bottle. We flew home the next day, Rovaniemi to Helsinki to London to Dublin. What a trek of a trip, but it was well worth it as the video captured all of the festive magic of Christmas and yet again we had another viral success on our hands.

Damo and Ivor were now known as comedy legends and Andy was getting mobbed everywhere we went. To cash in on the fame, the nightclub appearances came next. We hired legendary tour manager Marty Cullen and gigged all over Ireland and it was absolutely crazy. We decided it was best to do these appearances in character as Damo because he was the one for getting the crowd going. When people asked where Ivor was, we'd say his appearance fee was 150 grand so the club hadn't booked him and that always got a laugh. It was mad watching people meet Damo. They were hysterical. He signed knockers, bums and foreheads, all with permanent marker. Some girls were crying and screaming while the poor bouncers tried to keep everyone under control. In one club we had to take Damo out as there was such a crush of people it was getting dangerous. It was amazing to stand there and watch on as Damo performed the songs and see all the fans in the audience singing along. They knew all the words to songs we wrote. It blew me away at every gig we did.

Ruth in Parallel Pictures, with whom we had stayed in touch the whole time, saw the brand we had created and how popular it was. She arranged to meet us with

Eddie Doyle, the head of entertainment in RTÉ, to discuss creating a TV programme based around Damo and Ivor. Thankfully, Eddie had been following our progress and liked what we were doing. We whipped out the scripts and said, 'Ta dah! We're ready to rock!' So we applied to the Broadcasting Authority of Ireland to seek funding for our project. I had the candles lighting, the Buddha, Holy Mary and Padre Pio statues out. The smoke alarm was constantly going off due to all the incense I was burning. A couple of months later, we found out that our funding had been granted. I had always envisaged the moment of the news coming through and I thought I'd break down crying and shriek like I'd won the Lotto, but it was completely different when it actually happened. I couldn't speak. It took a full three weeks to sink in. This is it. We've got the production company, the funding, the broadcaster, they all believe in us. We've got the scripts, the fan base, everything. Holy shit. Three years of work is coming together and at the same time we haven't even started yet.

Before filming, Andy was in total lockdown preparing for the show. The double vodka and greasy kebab weekends were replaced with him jogging across Dublin like Forrest Gump, while I of course was still eating crap and relying on Red Bulls to be my diesel. The only exercise I was doing was squatting to look for food in the bottom of the fridge. We were both dying to get out there, on set, and start making our dream a reality. Working with Andy is amazing and without sounding like a big sap, I'm honoured that he let me in to share his dream with him. We've formed a powerful duo and it is true when they say it takes two to make a dream come true. Every sacrifice was worth it. The no wages being the hardest. Everything we made went straight back in to make more videos and songs. Thanks to modern piracy, you may have No. 1 singles on iTunes and an album out in the shops, but you make very little money from it. The memories for me will be the scraping together of cash to make music videos and finding dosh to go on the piss to destress afterwards. Days of having empty pockets and raiding the coin jar to pay for pizza to cure our hangovers. And my God, did we eat a lot of pizza and chipper food. My blood type was garlic dip.

While Andy had managed to get himself shredded in just a few weeks because he knew he had to do a topless sex scene, my latest attempt to lose weight had failed yet again. Just for the laugh, we had written in a small speaking part for me as the character DJ Deirdre. I needed to lose seven stone in two weeks, which was, of course, an impossible task, so I just thought, 'Feck it, I'll roll with it and be the fat skanger.' I wore a men's navy tracksuit with white stripes down the sleeves, a gold chain, gold onion-ring earrings and

I scraped my gelled hair up into a severe ponytail for that signature rough look. The scene was short. It was me miming to 'Ave Maria' while Damo and Ivor's grandmother, Grano, who was convinced she was dying, road-tested her flat-pack coffin from IKEA as I sang beside her and then asked her, 'So obviously I'm gettin' paid BEFORE da gig, yeah?' When I watched myself back on screen, I was horrified by what I saw. At 17 stone and dress size 18/20, I knew I was big and that the Deirdre look was unflattering, but I looked gigantic. My face looked like a basketball with make-up on it. Instead of this bald fact getting me down and maybe even pushing me to make changes, I yet again managed to shove the feelings somewhere deep into the pit of despair that lay inside me. I closed the lid and told myself that it wasn't me, it was DJ Deirdre who was massive. She was a whole other character. If you went on telly as yourself, you wouldn't look that big, Jules, the look is just unflattering and that's good for Deirdre, so just ignore the upset you feel and have a nice bar of chocolate to make yourself feel better. Yeah, that's a good idea. Jules in denial, yet again.

The night the series launched was spine-tingling. It was 25 September 2013. RTÉ 2 had mounted its biggest ever promotional campaign for a show and there were posters of *Damo & Ivor* on billboards, bus stops and advertising posts all over the country. The ad was playing on the radio and TV around the clock and I don't think there was a person in the country who wasn't aware that it was starting on Monday nights and would run for six weeks. I had watched all the episodes so many times by this stage that I had no interest in watching it when it was going out live. What I wanted to see was the social media reaction. I set up three computer screens in the office so I could see the tweets and comments as they trickled in. My desk looked like the Starship Enterprise. As soon as the ad break before the show came on, there were so many tweets pouring down the screen and at such speed, my eyeballs couldn't keep up with them. By the next ad break, we were trending No. 1 in Ireland on Twitter. The feedback was overwhelmingly amazing. We had delivered. This was the comedy Ireland had been gagging for. There were a lot of 'This is the best thing since *Father Ted*' messages. No higher compliment in our eyes. RTÉ, of course, were thrilled. Their most important measure is the audience figures and let's just say, we broke records. A second series was commissioned and we began writing immediately. I'm not an actor and even though I looked like a human JCB, I'd enjoyed my little Deirdre cameos in series one, DJing in the background of scenes. Visually I looked funny. Funny, but fat. So I vowed that I was going to lose weight and be a slim DJ Deirdre for series two. Sure I'd have loads of time to do it, I thought to myself. Grand.

I think people go one way or the other when it comes to motivation. I was on my healthy buzz with my latest fad diet. Nothing but rice cakes and tinned tuna with ten cups of green tea a day and a shot of wheatgrass, which I was even growing on the window ledge and juicing myself. On the *Damo & Ivor* Facebook page we announced a Hallowe'en fancy-dress competition, asking fans to submit photos of themselves pimped out like Damo or Ivor. We received hundreds of entries and the effort people went to was incredible. One picture sent in was a group of friends dressed up as the main characters: Damo, Ivor, Grano, Tracey, Spuddy and someone had done themselves up as DJ Deirdre. My heart sank when I looked at the photo. The thin girl had stuffed a pillow down the front of her tracksuit top in an attempt to make herself look as enormous as me. I threw the rice cakes in the bin and made myself a sandwich. You see, this is what I mean about people going one way or the other. I wish I was one of those people who would see that photo and make it be the turning-point, where they'd stand up and say, 'Right, that's it. I am determined to make a change.' Just like my grandfather did. He was a pioneer of the film industry who was told at an early age that he 'would only be a two-bit mechanic'. He set out to prove them wrong. I was the opposite. Moments like this always made me shatter and crumble to pieces and fall back into the Big Black Hole, yet again. And there I would stay, feeling hopeless and sorry for myself.

Just me, my inner bad bitch Siobhan and victimhood sitting in the darkness, eating.

Siobhan would tell me, 'You vat of lard. You obviously know this junk food you're eating is making things worse?' and I'd reply in my head, 'I know. I know. But just give me a few more days on it and then, when I get my strength back, I'll get back to the healthy stuff.' I didn't. And then it was Christmas and I spent the month with one hand in a tin of Roses and the other holding a glass of Baileys and a mince pie (I have big hands). And then it was January 2014 and inevitably, I started my New Year's resolutions full of gusto. Like always, I lasted for a mere week before being seduced again by my on-off boyfriend, chocolate.

I liken my relationship with chocolate to that of someone stuck in a domestic abuse relationship. Strong words, I know, but that's what it felt like. Except I was the one beating myself up. I blamed the chocolate for beguiling me. It would make me feel great for a few minutes and then the excess sugar would be converted to fat and my thighs would expand further and make me feel worse. And I'd torture myself mentally for being so weak. Why couldn't I walk away from chocolate? It felt like having a boyfriend who told me he loved me deeply, the sex with him was incredible, yet he would beat me daily. Who would stay in a relationship like that?

And yet in this imaginary relationship I had, there was nobody else involved. Chocolate is inanimate. Chocolate wasn't to blame. I was doing all of this to myself through the voices in my head. Those stupid, stupid voices. My stupid voice. Me. I wish I came with a button to restore myself back to factory settings. Sigh.

The best thing that came from *Damo & Ivor* was that I got to tick the No. 1 thing on my bucket list: I got to work with my ultimate hero and absolute love of my life. Not only that, I got to tick the second thing on my bucket list: shagging him. Well, I half-ticked it. Let me tell you about the greatest three days of my life ...

You always remember your first love, don't you? Towards the end of primary school lots of the girls in my class were kissing boys. I had still yet to talk to one as I didn't know how. I admired them from afar and I knew I'd like to kiss one, but at that stage I was so shy around anything with a willy that I would just watch on as my friends flirted their way around summer camp. When I was 12, the BBC aired a TV show called *Bottom* and from the very first episode I was in love with Rik Mayall, who would have been 33 at the time. Alongside fellow comedy genius Adrian Edmondson, they played the characters of Richie and Eddie, two hapless losers who lived in squalor and their main aim in life was to try and get a shag, but they perpetually failed. The script was littered with toilet humour, innuendos and comedy violence as they whacked each other over the head with frying pans. I couldn't get enough of it. Barry and I would watch the episodes over and over and fall around laughing. It drove Dad mad. 'What are you watching that garbage again for?' he'd ask. 'Dad, did you not just see Richie fall down the stairs and land head-first in the loo? It's hysterical!' And Dad would just roll his eyes and leave the room. He was more of an *Only Fools and Horses* kind of guy. I was all about *Bottom*.

I'd never been so enraptured by a television programme and that was entirely down to the fact that I'd discovered Rik. Now bear in mind that in the show he wore a white shirt and brown tie, blue jeans and a stupendously large pair of stained underpants that protruded from the top of his trousers and came up past his belly button. God, he was mad. I was head over heels watching his zany antics. He was so bold, you could see what he was thinking. Adrian was funny too, but I was just besotted with Rik. He was a big sweaty mess as he put so much effort into his performance and I loved him for it. He was unpredictable, clownish and just completely bonkers. My perfect man. I had never been so magnetically attracted to someone and I haven't since. Throughout my teenage years, my obsession continued. I watched all of his back catalogue and learned everything I possibly could about him personally and my love deepened. People would say to me, 'He's a great comedian, but you mean you actually fancy him, fancy him, like you'd kiss him?' Kiss him? I would snog every square millimetre of his beautiful face and body and shag him until his knob fell off if I got the chance!

When we were writing the first series of *Damo & Ivor*, we started envisioning who we'd like to play certain characters. We made a list and printed out pictures of the actors and stuck them up on the walls around us for inspiration. We named it 'The Wall of Attraction' as this would project out to the universe who we wanted to play the parts and energetically that would reel them in. We wondered who could play Ivor's posh, nasty bastard father. While writing the first scene, where Ivor is demanding cash from his moneybags parentals, Andy turned to me and said, 'You know who'd be great as Ivor's dad? Rik Mayall!' My eyes widened and my heart skipped a beat. How in the name of Greek buggery hadn't I thought of that?! My breathing quickened as I thought about the prospect. Imagine getting to meet him. Imagine WORKING with him?! 'Print out a picture of him quick!' I said to Andy. 'He needs to go up on The Wall so we can make this happen!' I couldn't work for the rest of the day as my mind was enthralled by the thoughts of Rik playing a part in a script that we had written. I was absolutely 100% categorically going to make this happen. There had never been a previous opportunity in my life to meet him and now this was it, and I was going for it.

When the time for casting came around, we told Ruth about our hopes and dreams for certain actors to play the parts. This wish list was sent on to our amazing casting director, Louise Kiely. It was a highly aspirational line up, including Ruth McCabe from *The Snapper* and *My Left Foot* for the part of Grano. She was the key actor we were hoping to secure. And then we mentioned Rik Mayall. My only fear was that we couldn't afford him. I had read in his autobiography about a commercial he did in the 1990s for Super Nintendo and he made so much money from it, he bought a mansion and aptly named it 'Nintendo Towers'. But this was a decade on and since his very serious quad bike accident, which had nearly killed him, he hadn't done a huge amount of television work. So I figured there was a sliver of a chance that he might actually be amenable to our madcap idea. However, our casting director thought it a seriously long shot for another reason: Ivor's father only appeared in the first episode and then absconded in the second. I begged her to at least try and see if we could get him, thinking to myself, 'He's probably way out of budget, but if we don't ask, we'll never know.'

The script was sent to Rik's agent and we waited with bated breath. I kept up my positive visualisations in my head, day-dreaming all day long of Rik being on set, speaking the words of our script. I also had plenty of sexy fantasies too, of course, where I'd dream that I was a size 10 temptress, wearing a low-cut red dress with my jugs pouring out the front of it and I'd imagine myself seducing Rik with my fantastic knockers and witty banter and him ravaging me round the back of the make-up trailer and telling me, as he shagged my brains out, that he was divorcing his wife immediately and going to spend the rest of his waking life rogering me senseless. Sigh. I knew he was happily married and that could never happen, but a girl can dream, can't she?

A few days later Louise phoned and I remember standing up out of my chair to receive the news. 'I'm really sorry, Jules, but it's a no from Rik,' she delicately told me, knowing it was crushing my heart like a butcher's meat hammer. 'What?!' I retorted. 'No way. This isn't how it's meant to go. No, no, no. I've already felt that it's going to happen. My intuition has been telling me he's going to do it. How can this be? Why did he say no? Is it money? Is he way out of budget? We can move the budget around and take money from my writing fees to pay him. Will that work? Or does he want mega-money?' I desperately questioned.

'Jules, his agent said he was thankful to be considered for the role and he thought the scripts were great and very funny but his reason for turning it down was just that the role was too small as he's only in the first episode.'

'Well, we didn't think we'd be able to afford him for more than a few days' filming, so that's all we could fit him in for in the script.'

'I know. I'm so sorry, Jules, but don't worry, we'll find another great actor for the part.'

After finishing up the call, you'd think I'd slump back into my chair, crushed, but no, my instinct to fight the rejection was so strong I absolutely point-blank refused to accept this fate. Somewhere inside my core, I was certain he was going to play the part. I could see it in the future. I just knew.

After pacing around furiously, chain-smoking fags and discussing it at length with Andy, who also felt the same instinct, I decided that I was going to write to Rik to see if I could persuade him to say yes. I mean, if I could convince Mum to let me go to discos as a teenager, surely I could do this? Louise wasn't too keen on the idea of me writing to Rik, but I told her that while I appreciated there was etiquette she had to obey as the casting director dealing with agents, we now had nothing to lose. I requested that she blame any possible aftermath entirely on me outrageously breaking all protocol, because I knew Rik would do the same if he was in my boots. Thankfully, Louise succumbed and said she'd send on the letter to his agent once I'd written it. Knowing I was the Mayall worshiper that I am, Andy left me to it and I locked myself in the office for two hours and delicately constructed the ultimate letter of persuasion. I wanted Rik to read it and know that not only was I a fan of his but that I was a life-long hardcore fan who had read his autobiography, *Bigger Than Hitler. Better Than Christ*, from cover to cover umpteen times. I have a Masters degree in Rik. So there are a few references in this composition that you might not get, unless you're a Mayall maniac like me, but they were designed to make Rik chuckle.

Here is the letter I sent.

> Dearest The Rik Mayall,
>
> Thank you for your kind words about our scripts. We are honoured that a pan global phenomenon such as yourself has read and enjoyed them. There is no greater compliment in our eyes!
>
> We are Jules and Andy – the writers and producers of *Damo & Ivor* and Andy plays the parts of both main characters. We are

devastated (that's the strongest word we could find in the dictionary, but we still don't think it covers it) to hear that you've turned down the role of Alistair Itchdaddy. We understand and appreciate your reasons for doing so, but the desolation is so unbearable that we have decided to break all protocol and send a heartfelt plea to see if we can sway your beautiful mind.

We are HUGE, actually what's a bigger word than huge? *consults thesaurus* GIGANTIC admirers of you and your incredible accomplishments in comedy, acting and just being an all-round legend, and a very handsome one at that we might add! We have followed your success for a long time. It really is hard to believe that you've achieved as much as you have when they say your career has spanned 40 years – how is that possible when you don't look a day over 39? There really must be something in that salad cream moisturiser! You should bottle it!

Anyway, back to the plea (please imagine us with big puppy dog eyes as you read this). We'll never forget the day we laughed for the first time. We were in our early teens and *Bottom* came onto our TV screens. We still quote lines from it on a daily basis. If there's a knock on the door and I say 'Who is it?', Andy will always reply 'It's the gas man!' We grew up watching it and know all the episodes inside out. It's still our favourite TV show.

We started writing *Damo & Ivor* three years ago and it has been an epic journey. We have made huge sacrifices, taken risks and worked our bollixes off to get where we are today. This is the first thing we've ever written and the first thing Andy has acted in and everything is going so well we feel like we're riding around on unicorns and farting rainbows. The fanbase is huge and RTÉ, our national broadcaster, is already talking about a second series, which is bloody brilliant, hence our desire to establish Ivor with the right father from the start.

If we had known that you would have even considered the role of Alistair, we would have written him into all six episodes, but the story was such that we had to make bad things happen to Ivor for the sake of the funnies and take his 'ATM' away from him and hence the Alistair and the Criminal Assets Bureau storyline. We wanted to tell you that if we do a second series and we had you on board from series one, we would definitely make Alistair a lead role in series two and give you shit loads of jokes and killer lines to deliver.

We just know you'd do an incredible job playing Alistair. So if you take a chance on us and be our Alistair it would be the greatest thing that could happen to us, the show and let's be honest, the world!

So in summary, Rik Tripod Mayall, please accept our impassioned plea to be Alistair Itchdaddy and share your wondrous talents with Ireland.

Sincerely yours (and we mean that in every sense, if you'd like a shag or a blow job thrown in as part of the deal, just say!),

Jules & Andy

Of course I was fully prepared to be the face of that sexy offer should he have wanted it included in the bargain. Sadly, he didn't. I was ill with anticipation for the next 24 hours, constantly looking at my phone, waiting for a call from Louise. Finally it came.

'Jules, your letter worked! Rik's going to play the part!'

'AAAAAAAAAGGGGHHHHH!!!!' bellowed from my ecstatic lungs as loudly as it would if I'd just rolled deodorant on my freshly shaven armpits. Andy was jumping around the place and I always thought at a moment like this that I'd be swept away in a wave of emotion and start bawling my eyes out, but I didn't. I just felt sheer joy and shock at the same time, not realising that the reality of it wasn't actually going to hit home until I came face to face with Rik, in the flesh.

They say you should never meet your heroes. Well, that's only true if you have a shit hero and in that case, you deserve it. Rik was my hero and he was fucking amazing! On the final week of filming, he flew in the day before he was due to shoot. We had arranged to meet him in the lobby of the Beacon Hotel, where he was staying. It was the most surreal moment of my life. Part of me feared that it was all a prank and that someone was going to jump out and say, 'Ha! Jules! You didn't really think Rik was coming, did you? You twat!' I received a text from Ruth, our producer, to say that she was with Rik and our director, Rob, and they were sitting in the lobby beside the front entrance. Andy and I walked in nervously and I remember laying eyes on Rik and finally knowing that it wasn't all a spoof. He was there. My hero. My idol. The unadulterated love of my life. Sitting right there. I placed my hand on Andy's arm and looked at him. 'This is it, Teddy. I'm gonna meet Rik.' Andy's eyes dazzled with excitement for both of us. I don't think my feet touched the ground as we approached the table. Rik stood up. His grey hair rested magnificently on his broad shoulders and he was even bigger and more solid in the flesh than I had imagined. Be still, my beating clitoris.

Rik was introduced to Andy and they shook hands with vigour and then he turned to me. I blurted out, 'I can't believe this. I feel like I should curtsy!', which I duly did and Rik laughed. Bloody hell. Rik Mayall just laughed at words that came out of my mouth. Cupid has left the building; his work here is done. We all sat down and I can't remember anything that was discussed initially as I was absolutely hypnotised by the gargantuan aura of charisma that Rik projected. I've never come across anything like it in my life, and Andy said the same afterwards. Rik was resplendent in every sense. Such a gentleman, so witty and so flippin' gorgeous. I should have brought a towel to sit on. We chatted for two hours and after Ruth and Rob left, Andy and I ended up smoking fags outside with Rik for another hour, talking about all sorts. His ability to tell a story was phenomenal and we were laughing so much I felt bereft of ribs. I think he warmed to us too, as he really seemed to be enjoying himself. All the while I'm thinking, 'God, I hope there's batteries in my vibrator when I get home.'

The following day on set, Rik filmed his first scene as Ivor's prick of a father, Alistair Itchdaddy. He told us he loved the part as 'playing a complete bastard' was his favourite thing to do. After the first take, he stepped out of the room and said in quite a serious manner, 'Jules. Andy. Can I speak to you both in private, please?' Oh sweet Jesus. What's wrong? I anxiously walked over, believing he was going to say, 'This is shit. I'm not happy with the camera angle. This was all a mistake. Fuck you both. I'm going home.' But he didn't. Instead, he said, 'Are you happy with the way I performed that?' I immediately gushed, 'Oh my God, Rik, it was amazing! Perfec—' 'Jules,' he interrupted, 'I'm asking if you're happy with the way I've interpreted the character. As you are the writers, fuck the director, I want to know if this is how you had envisioned Alistair to be?' Wow. Not one other actor had asked us that. I think he knew from the look in my eyes how sincere I was when I smiled at him and gratefully said, 'Thank you, Rik. It's exactly how we imagined it.' 'Good,' he replied. 'Now if there's any part of my performance that's not in keeping with your vision, you're to tell me immediately, okay? You are the writers. This is your creation, remember!' And off he marched, back to the set for take two. Andy and I looked at each other wide-eyed. At this stage, I think Andy was nearly as in love with him as I was.

Now while I've had plenty of great days in my life, including the monumental day that I drove across three lanes of the M50 motorway without touching any cat's eyes, 3 May 2013 was, as it turns out, the absolute BEST day of my life. My wedding day and the birth of my first child might come a hair's breadth close to it, but I'll have to see when I meet my Mr Right (if he's reading this in the future, you've got a lot to live up to, mate!). While filming at the Leopardstown Racecourse, Rik was swanning around like a peacock in his pinstripe suit having a great time, enjoying the shoot. The paparazzi had arrived and Rik was happily throwing them the two fingers as they tried to nab pics. He was so charming, the whole crew were enamoured by him. Mum and Dad were there that day as extras and after chatting to Rik they were both completely taken by him. 'Now do you see why I've been so obsessed with him all these years?' I asked Dad, to which he laughed and said, 'I get it now, Jules, I get it now.' Andy and I experienced a magic moment while Rik was having his make-up done when he spontaneously burst into song, singing 'The Bare Necessities' from *The Jungle Book* and we all joined in. I was on cloud nine. Afterwards I knocked on his dressing-room door to ask him a favour. I presented him with two of my hardback copies of the scripts from *Bottom* and asked him would he mind signing them for me. He happily obliged and sat down, black marker in hand and wrote on the inside cover:

> This is for my number 1 bird Jules. She's MY
> bird ok?? So fucking lay off her everyone
> else right – no snogging, pants-offing or
> upstairs feeling* ok? (*jug fondling) Jules is
> MINE. BY LAW. Signed by Dr. The Fucking
> Rik Mayall ©

And he finished it off with ten kisses and underlined several of the words to emphasise them. This is now my prized possession and God forbid there was a fire in my gaff, this would be the first and only thing I would grab before jumping out the window.

Later that day, while they were filming scenes with Ivor, I wondered where Rik had disappeared to. I went outside to the balcony and then walked down the stairs. As I reached the bottom, his purr caressed my ears as I heard him say 'Helloooooo Jules' as only he can. His sumptuous voice was like a cello deep-fried in butter and drizzled in golden syrup. Startled, I turned to my right and there he was, casually smoking a cigarette. He gently patted the stool beside him, signalling for me to join him. He offered me one of his cigarettes, lit it for me and we chatted. This was my nirvana. 'I would finish you like a cheesecake,' I thought to myself while looking into his eyes. As we spoke, I can't even remember what we were talking about, while I was mid-sentence he put his hand on my arm and interrupted, 'Look!' He pointed up to the most spectacular rainbow I have ever witnessed, which was radiating across the sky above the racecourse. 'Wow!' I exclaimed. He turned and looked at me and said, 'This is really special. We'll always remember this moment.' How I didn't rip off all my clothes and pant 'Take me!', I don't know. Well, it's probably because I thought he might reply, 'Ugh. Put that flab away! No man could get a boner looking at all that cellulite!' Yet I know he would never say anything like that.

They were long days on set, with a lot of sitting around. One day, while I was busy surfing social media on my phone, Rik came over near me quietly singing to himself, 'I've got a big knob, such a big knob and I'm so in love with Jules ... Oh hi, Jules!' and he pretended he'd just noticed me sitting there. I laughed and whispered, 'How big is it?' He replied, 'Bigger than you could ever imagine!' I couldn't help playing along. 'Well, like, how big? An elephant's trunk? A giraffe's neck?' Rik interjected, 'No, no, no! Like a load of killer whales all sellotaped together! THAT BIG!' I fell around the place laughing. Seizing this opportune moment, I asked Ronan, our set photographer, if he'd take some photos of me with Rik. A high-res picture with Rik. Bucket list – tick! Susie, our lovely hairdresser, backcombed my hair for me (the bigger the hair, the smaller the face). I fixed my make-up and approached Rik with my request. 'Of course, my darling! Where's the photographer?'

Rik was animated in real life, but even more so as soon as there was a camera present. I had seen loads of bonkers funny photos online of him doing crazy poses with fans and I couldn't believe that it was now my turn. For the first photo, he put his arm around my shoulder and smiled sweetly as Ronan snapped away. 'Right, that's the nice one,' he said. Next, he gently cupped my right boob with his left hand. 'You don't mind, do you?' 'Not at all!' I exclaimed, laughing my head off while secretly thinking, 'He's touching my boob! Hashtag wank bank lodgement deposited!' Then he signalled for me to turn around. I wondered why. 'Turn around?' I asked. 'Turn around, Jules! Trust me!' So I turned my back to him and he swiftly grabbed a chair that was close by, put it in front of me and bent me over it, grasped a bunch of my hair in his hand and began humping me with a cartoonish expression on his face. I was in hysterics laughing and played along, putting my hand over my mouth and pretending to look shocked for the camera. THIS was the greatest moment of my life. All my dreams come true. Now of course actual shagging would have been even better, but I was happy to settle for a dry hump as it was as close as I was going to get. It still makes my heart flutter knowing that for that unforgettable 30 seconds there was just a bit of fabric separating our nether regions. *happy sigh*

I wondered how I was ever going to find another man who could make me feel like this. He was absolutely everything I wanted. At the wrap party that evening we had to say goodbye. He sidled up to me and said, 'Jules, I'm fucking starving so I'm going up to my room to order something. I don't want to do a big goodbye thing as it'll take me forever, so I'm going to sneak out.' He took both of my hands and held them and with, no joke, tears in his eyes he looked at me and told me how much he'd enjoyed working with us and playing the part of Alistair. He made me promise that we'd write him into all six episodes of the next series. I vowed that we would, and that we'd give him some of his favourite comedy violence too. We hugged and he slipped away through the crowd, leaving me the most satisfied girl on the planet.

In the following months, he would call every once in a while to say hello and text to check in on how the writing was going. His texts were always hilarious, with all sorts of obscene funny sign-offs, like 'With love and a big snog on the vagina, Rik xxx'. I still can't believe I became mates with my hero. We duly kept our promise and wrote his character Alistair into all of series two. We sent the scripts to Rik and he rang to say that he loved them and had been reading them to his kids, who'd been laughing their arses off. He couldn't wait to come over for filming. I was so excited about seeing him again.

Three weeks before we were due to start shooting, my brother Gavin phoned me. I answered, 'Hiya Teddy!' I could hear him breathing. 'Jules … Rik Mayall is dead.' 'What? Are you joking? Because if this is a joke, it is not funny!' I said. I could hear the trembling in Gavin's voice and I knew he was telling the truth. 'It's on the news. He died this morning.' I dropped the phone and ran to the kitchen with Andy to turn on the TV. I didn't believe it until I saw the Sky News ticker-tape scrolling on screen, confirming the horrific news that he had died from a sudden heart attack at the age of 56. I was devastated and absolutely inconsolable. I'm crying again now just remembering it. Within the hour, the press were on to us, looking for a statement and wondering what we were going to do as they knew he was going to be in series two. 'Fuck them all,' I told Andy. 'We are not giving a statement. I couldn't give a shite. Our friend has died. I can't think past that, let alone what we're going to do for the show.' When I'd composed myself later, and after discussing it with Ruth, we agreed that the only person we'd talk to was Ray D'Arcy on his radio show the following morning. We knew Ray would handle it with compassion and not pry as to what our solution for replacing Rik was going to be because obviously we didn't have one. So as a tribute to Rik, we went on air with Ray and talked about how tremendous Rik was and how much he meant to us. Later, Andy and I went to the

Beacon Hotel and sat at the same table, in the same seats as that fateful night we all first met. We ordered Rik a whiskey and set it out in front of his vacant chair and reminisced about the incredible time we got to spend with him.

In the coming days, as there was only three weeks before filming began, we had to decide what we were going to do without him. There was talk of replacing him with another actor, but Andy and I wouldn't hear of it. Rik was irreplaceable and I argued that even if we brought in Daniel Day-Lewis in prosthetic make-up, he still wouldn't be capable of being Rik. Moreover, as a mark of respect, Andy and I didn't want anyone else acting out the script that we had written specifically for him. So we stayed up night and day and changed the storyline and rewrote all the scenes he was in. It was totally worth the resulting eye-bags. Those were Rik's lines and nobody else was having them.

He is my first love and if my Mr Right is even a fragment of how fantastic Rik was, then I will be a very lucky girl. I still miss him and think about him often. I have the picture of us together framed beside my bed. My only regret is that I'm fat in the photo and I'll never get to have another photo taken with him now that I'm slim. But I know that I'm so lucky that he was part of my life. Part of me still won't accept that he's gone. But I take solace in the fact that they say if a writer falls in love with you, then you can never die.

In 2008 Rik was given an honorary doctorate from Exeter University. In his incredible speech he gave five mantras to carry with you through life, which he claimed had helped him not only to survive but to be happy. Here they are.

> All men are equal. Therefore no one can ever be your genuine superior.
>
> It is your future. It is yours to create. Your future is as bright as you make it.
>
> Change is a constant of life, so you must never lose your wisdom.
>
> If you want to live a full and complete life, you have to be free. Freedom is paramount.
>
> Love is the answer. Love IS the answer.

Rik told his audience of students to 'make sure you've got those five things. Equality, opportunity, wisdom, freedom and love, and you'll be alright.'

Before now, nobody but Rik and his agent had read that letter I sent him asking him to accept the part. When it came time to promoting *Damo & Ivor* and the press enquired as to how we managed to get the legendary Rik Mayall to be in the show, we told them that he loved the scripts and it was as simple as that. We didn't want to say it took a begging letter, but now that Rik has passed, I don't think he'd mind me sharing it as a good example of grabbing life by the balls and going for it, especially as nobody liked a good gonad grabbing more than Rik.

On the first day of filming series two, I asked Rik to send me a sign that he was with us in spirit, looking over us. The day was glorious and the sun was beaming, but soon after I put out my request to Rik it quickly changed to grey skies and the heavens opened. I dashed to my back-pack and pulled out my raincoat. The last time I'd worn it was while we were filming series one, the previous year. As I stood in the rain, waiting for the first shot to be set up, I put my hand in the pocket of my raincoat and pulled out a keyring with a photo of Rik on it. It had fallen off my keys last year while filming and I had put it in my pocket for safe-keeping but then forgot about it. That, along with the glorious rainbow that shortly afterwards appeared in the sky, were my signs that Rik was with me in spirit. Ever since then, I talk to him regularly as I know his presence is around me. I call him in every day as I write this book and I ask him to help me. I picture him just like he was in *Drop Dead Fred*, when he played the naughty imaginary friend. I know he's still with me, even if it's just in spirit, and that's good enough for me.

I didn't manage to lose any weight by the time we'd started filming series two. Quite the opposite. I was now 34 years old and weighed 19 stone, but I was completely unaware of this fact as I had not stepped on the scales for fear of what I'd see on the dial. I was in the dangerous red section of the body mass index chart because I was now 'morbidly obese'. And it's hardly surprising when I was guzzling Red Bulls and living on a diet of baguette rolls, crisps and bars, every intake looking like a Hungry Hungry Hippos game. My sugary diet made my face so bloated that my eyes, nose and mouth looked like they were protruding through a pillow. I felt so big that I was sure I had my own solar system. Siobhan now rabbited in my ear 24 hours a day. Her voice consumed me as she constantly and continually reminded me of how fat, ugly and horrible I looked.

Filming series two, I donned my leopard-print pyjama bottoms and zip-up hoodie to play DJ Deirdre again. We had written in a few scenes with a speaking part for me, just for the craic. The first scene we filmed was DJ Deirdre walking in the back door of Grano's gaff with a massive hangover after a hen night. When I watched back the take and saw the size of my face and enormous double chin, I was horrified. It was the size of the feckin' moon. Siobhan wondered, 'Jesus, Jules, how can it even get any bigger? Maybe someday soon your head is just going to explode like a cartoon?'

I was so sweaty all the time, even just standing around. So I religiously kept a hairband in my handbag and would put it on to soak up the sweat from my head and prevent it running down my face. What I really needed was a sweat band like John McEnroe wore. I also used to put Driclor, a really strong antiperspirant, on my forehead to try and prevent the embarrassment of my drippy face. I was so conscious of it that when I was in a conversation with someone and I could feel the beads gathering on my forehead, like a tiara made from sweat instead of diamonds, I employed some (rehearsed) slick moves to casually wipe my forehead with my hand and not make it look like I was mopping my brow. I was just nonchalantly flicking my hair or putting my hand on my forehead for dramatic effect.

Every move I made took such great effort because I had so much extra mass to cart around. I'd remember the days of being able to get up from the sofa without having to make sound effects. Good times. My thighs rubbed together like sandpaper with every step, so much so my size 22 jeans would have friction holes in the crotch and I'd have to bin them on a regular basis. I found it increasingly difficult to find clothes to fit me. The plus-size shops, like Evans, went up to a size 32, but I thought their clothes really dowdy and unflattering. They were all covered in big prints and that made me look even bigger. Good auld Marks & Spencer went up to a size 28, so I did most of my black uniform shopping in there. I never even went into any high-street stores like River Island or Oasis as I'd only be teasing myself with the fabulously fashionable clothes available for slim people. My boobs were flippin' gigantic. I was only short of putting my bra on with a boomerang as my circumference was now so big. I was wearing a size 44E bra and putting a bra-extender clip, sometimes even two, on the back of it to give myself more room to breathe. The poor underwire was under such a burden it would forever try to break free and pop out and stab me in the chest for putting it under such stress.

I had been hiding from exercise in the fitness protection programme. Well, I did five sit-ups every morning. That might not sound like much, but there's only so many times you can hit the snooze button. I knew I needed to get in shape as if I was murdered right then, the chalk outline would be a circle. The only part of my body that was actually exercising was the hamster on the wheel in my head. He was like Usain Bolt, pegging it along as the negative thoughts about my body churned in my mind. I'd say 90% of my thinking was about my weight. And my daydreams about being skinny were always interrupted by the sound of my own chewing. I was in a constant state of panic. Things had gone so far now, I didn't know what to do. Siobhan would incessantly berate me with abuse as I looked in the mirror, telling me, 'You are so fat. You look disgusting. Look at those rolls of blubber. You are vile, you lard-arse fat pig.' And of course, thoughts become things, so by the law of attraction all I was doing was making myself fatter. But I just couldn't get my thoughts under control and the only time Siobhan could be muted was while I was eating, so that's what I would do. As soon as I was done, Siobhan grabbed her megaphone and turned the volume up to 11 and abused me by telling me how guilty I should feel for eating what I just ate.

I had planned on losing weight before going on camera to film *Damo & Ivor*, but the task was so monumental that I had epically failed by not even attempting to try. But then came the day when I realised what it was all about. I'll have to rewind a bit first and build up to my big moment of revelation.

I remember when I was growing up, Mum was so frustrated with Barry because his bedroom was always so messy: piles of clothes all over the floor, cereal bowls stacked up, bed never made, etc. Barry wasn't lazy though, as in all other aspects of his life he was a high achiever. He is quite the little genius and is so highly intelligent, he's the guy you'd always want on your team at a table quiz. If a question came up like 'What is chewing gum made of?' Barry would be the guy who'd know that 'It's made from chicle that comes from the sapodilla tree'. We call him 'Information Desk' as he just knows bleedin' everything! Mum would nag him constantly to clean his room, but it remained a perpetual scattered mess. Then one day, after watching a segment on *Oprah* about perfectionists, it suddenly hit Mum that that's what Barry was: a perfectionist! Her discovery from the show was that for a perfectionist there is a perfect place for everything and if the perfectionist doesn't have the time to find that place or know where that 'perfect spot' is, then they'll put things anywhere rather than risk failing. So while Barry would actually like to have his room neat and orderly, because it would never be 'perfect' according to his standards, he let it go the other way because the perfection was unattainable.

We got another insight into perfection while watching a TV show called *Child Genius* on Channel 4. There was a boy named Dante, aged 11, and he was visiting Joan, a child psychologist, for an IQ test. This was their conversation.

Joan: Disproportionate?

Dante: Disproportionate is where it's meant to be the same but they're totally different scales of magnitude.

Joan: Ochre?

Dante: Ochre is known as earth blood. It's a red dye that comes from clay.

Joan: Perfect. Repose?

Dante: I'm sorry, but I'm just totally lost.

Joan: Believe me, nobody finishes these tests.

Dante: I don't want to embarrass myself.

Joan: Do you aim to be perfect all the time?

Dante: I think it's good to be perfect.

Joan: Doesn't it cause a lot of trouble?

Dante: Well, it causes a lot of energy to be spent, but in the end perfection is the aim of any person who wants to create anything, isn't it?

Joan: Well, how do you know when you've reached perfection if you are creating something, like painting a picture?

Dante: Painting a picture? When you have achieved your goal in every way.

Joan: But how do you know when you've achieved your goal? How do you know that one slap of paint more wouldn't be better?

Dante: You never do. That's why perfection is impossible. You can only reach perfection in imperfection. Like, that wouldn't be the absolute most perfect IQ test ever conceived, but if you got every answer right you would have a perfect score.

Joan: Yes.

Dante: So you can only reach perfection in a frame of imperfection.

Joan: Very philosophical.

Dante: Yay for me! I've redeemed myself!

Joan: (interview to camera) Dante is a great character. He's got a fantastic wit. His problems are that he somehow has the feeling of not being quite good enough and that's why he's aiming for perfection. Whereas in fact he IS quite good enough but he just doesn't feel it somehow and this puts quite a burden on him, because nobody can be perfect and so he must fail and it's that fear of failure which dogs you throughout life.

Well, when Mum and I watched this we paused it, looked at each other with our mouths hanging open and then we rewound it and watched it again several times in a row. Firstly, we couldn't believe such philosophical genius was coming from the mouth of an 11-year-old child, but mainly we were blown away by this revelation about perfection. It is so true. We are all striving for the unattainable and thus we can only fail as the goal we seek doesn't even exist. For some people that means 'If I can't be a best-selling author, I won't write a word', 'If I can't run as fast as the person next to me, I get off the treadmill', 'If I can't decorate my house just like the pictures in glossy magazines, I won't put anything on the walls.' And then it gets worse: 'If I can't have the perfect house, I'll live in a cluttered mess', 'If I can't be the perfect size, I'll stuff my face', 'If I can't be the fastest and the best and the most perfect and the brightest and the shiniest and the most beautiful, I just won't do any of it.' Perfectionists *want* to be the best, but they don't want to work at something that they might not ever achieve. Because the threat of failure is too much to bear.

I applied the Oprah and Dante slants to my weight and realised that that was exactly what I'd been doing. I wanted a perfect body, but because I feared that I wouldn't be able to achieve that goal, instead I accelerated in the opposite direction. I had become perfectly fat instead of perfectly slim. Mum and I sat and talked openly about the solution for this mode of thinking. What do we aim for instead of 'perfection'? We concluded that our new goal for everything was going to be 'good enough'. That was the new aim of the game.

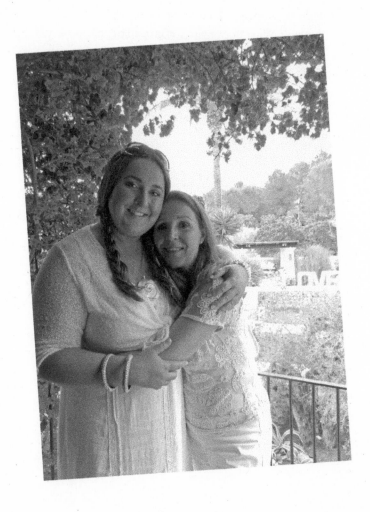

# 7

# Fat Girl Slim

'Coming up after the break. Meet the woman who lost 300 pounds and transformed her life!'

I'd eagerly grab a cup of tea and some chocolate (obvs) and sit down to watch. Weight-loss TV shows were my favourite. I'd always cry watching them, when I'd see the person shed the pounds and be free from being trapped in an obese body. Half of me was crying because I was so happy for them and the other half of me, the fat half, was crying because I was so envious that they'd done it. I watched these shows all the time, looking for inspiration and searching for answers. 'How had they done it? Were they a guinea pig for a new miracle pill that some ride of a scientist had invented? Were they going to wrap themselves in cling-film and then put on a waist trainer and sit in a sauna? Has that been done before?' I wondered. I was sure there had to be an easy way. But as I watched show after show and saw countless people shrink, I realised that there were three common denominators in all of the success stories and that they were pretty simple. No. 1: They all quit eating junk food and started eating healthily 24/7. No. 2: They all exercised. No. 3: They all made sacrifices and resisted slipping back into their old ways as they now realised that this was a change of lifestyle, not a diet. This was going to be their new way of life, for life. 'For feck's sake! C'mon, diet industry! Will you not invent an easy solution that actually feckin' works?! Or do you just want us to all stay fat and addicted so we continue to spend all our money on packaged foods and drinks and then get more obese and sick and then spend all our money on pharmaceutical drugs?!' ... Ermagawd. I realised that's exactly what they want. We all get fat and sick and they get fat wallets.

One thing that really stood out for me in watching these weight-loss candidates on TV is that each of them had a pretty evident emotional issue, aka their 'sob story', which was documented in the programme.

They had all suffered some sort of trauma, such as grief, divorce, a miscarriage, bullying, a bad relationship break-up, abuse, a traumatic childhood … The list was endless. Now I ain't no psychiatrist, but I could see it plain as natural yogurt that all of their excess weight was emotional baggage with a root cause.

And that made me think, 'What sort of suitcases of sadness am I carrying around with me? If all these pounds are problems, then what's my problem?' I couldn't think of anything. I've been lucky enough in this incarnation to have lived a charmed life. It's been wonderful. I've wanted for nothing. I haven't suffered. The only thing that's shite in my life is the fact that I'm fat, but that's the effect, not the cause. I racked my brains. 'Is it because you've never had a boyfriend?' I asked myself. 'But I don't have one because I'm fat. I could easily bag one if I was slim,' I told myself. 'Okay, so then trace it back. When did you start to put on weight?' I thought about it and knew that it was since that summer in Ios, when I was 19. 'Okay, so what happened in Ios that would trigger 15 years of weight gain?' I asked myself. 'I had the time of my life in Ios! It was great! Yeah, I got hauled home for the credit card bill, but that was grand and I paid it back.' I was left blank. I couldn't figure it out. I considered myself to be a happy person in general, just unhappy about my weight.

So I went back to the doc and I asked him to send me to a psychiatrist for an emotional lobotomy. I figured that if I couldn't work out what was wrong with my head, then surely a professional could. He sent me to St Patrick's Mental Hospital, to the eating disorders unit. 'Eh sorry, what? Is that not for people with anorexia and bulimia?' I wondered. Then I realised that obesity and over-eating is just as much of an eating disorder as the other end of the scale. At St Pat's I met a lovely psychiatrist who spent two hours picking through my life and analysing me. I was brutally honest and open in all of my answers to her questions because I desperately wanted her to figure me out and tell me what was wrong inside my head. But at the end of the session she couldn't figure out an emotional cause to my weighty issues. 'So you're not going to put me in a strait-jacket?' I enquired. 'No, we're not. I'm going to send you in to the doctor to discuss the medical side of things.' After I'd seen the doctor, she chatted to the psychiatrist and then I was brought in and told that it seemed that my PCOS and hormonal imbalance seem to be the main cause of my obesity. The stupid frickin' hormones *were* to blame. Those shaggin' little bastards!

Back to the doc.

'Right, so the shrink can't find any emotional cause behind my weight. I thought if I could find one, then

I could heal it and my body wouldn't have to reflect those issues back to me. But seeing as I haven't been committed, I now want to look into my next option, weight-loss surgery. I have struggled for 15 years and I'm continuing to spiral out of control. So today I am finally admitting that I can't do this by myself. I need help. I need an intervention. A drastic one.'

I had been researching weight-loss surgery online and learning everything I possibly could about it. I even watched the gory operations on YouTube. The before and after photos were phenomenal. 'I want to be one of those transformations,' I thought to myself. I was so, so tired of being fat. It was a huge step for me to ask for help. Normally I am very independent – in fact, I'm a control freak. It drives me bonkers in the supermarket when I see that they have people there packing up your groceries in exchange for a donation to their charity. I just stand there thinking, 'Thank you, amateur bag-packer, for packing my shopping in such a nonsensical way considering that all of the items were grouped on the conveyor belt in an orderly fashion,' as they pile the two litres of milk on top of the carton of eggs. Sigh.

If you want a job done right, do it yourself, isn't that what they say? With most things in life I can achieve my goal, but now, for the first time, I had to admit that I couldn't do this alone. I needed professional help to intervene and help me solve my big problem. Of course, the first thing that crossed my mind should have been: 'Will I live to tell the tale? Surgery comes with risks and possible complications. Are you willing to risk your life to be slim?' But no, that wasn't my first thought. It was: 'How much is this going to cost?' That was my main concern. I googled and googled, but there wasn't much information about prices online. From the little data I did find on the web, I figured I was looking at about 15 to 20 thousand smackers. Holy shiteballs on a stick. Where in the name of size 10 Victoria's Secret knickers was I going to get that?! Because I certainly didn't have it. I had reached a point in my life, career-wise, where I was doing well, certainly not minted, but well. *Damo & Ivor* was going to fund my surgery, I decided, so I worked my ass off and I started saving every penny I made. In the meantime, I decided I was going to learn everything I possibly could about bariatric surgery, up to the point where I could nearly perform the operation myself, even under anaesthetic.

As I researched online, I saw that there were cheaper options available than getting it done in Ireland. You could fly to Belgium and have a gastric band for five K. 'Oooooh! Belgium! They make amazing chocolates!' I thought. But as I looked into it further, there were numerous horror stories from previous patients warning not to do it as they had the surgery and were then turfed out of the hospital after 24 hours and left to recover in a grotty B&B, and then had to endure the abysmal experience of flying home just after having a serious operation. I shut the laptop and asked myself, 'Jules, are you booking a holiday here? Eh, no. Then what are you doing even thinking of looking into getting it done on the cheap?! This is a life-changing intervention. You need to engage Dad's mantra: *If you're going to do it, do it right.*' And that's what I did. Dad's a great man for that. If there's a household appliance, a car or the likes to be bought, he'll do his research and find the best quality and the best price and then save up and purchase the best and then it lasts for years and years, instead of buying the cheapest option that falls apart and has to be replaced over and over. So I wrote off the idea of the yellow-pack surgery as my intuition just told me it wasn't the right direction for me to go. Instead, I visited a private hospital in Dublin. It was going to cost a fat arm and a fat leg and it might take me a good while to save up for it, but I was going to value myself enough to go to the best surgeon and hospital our country had to offer to ensure that I was in the safest of hands.

I was very excited about my first consultation. I met the bariatric surgeon in his office and immediately liked him and his gentle manner. I spied the weighing scales in the corner of the room. It was industrial and looked like it could weigh a farm animal. 'I haven't been on the scales in a good while, but I think I'm around 17 stone or so,' I told him. I stepped onto the sad step and closed my eyes as the number shot up. He told me I weighed 120 kg and jotted it down. '120 kilos? I'm still on the stone-age system. What's that in pounds?' I asked. 'That's 266 pounds,' he said. I tried to divide that by 14 in my head. Now I wished I'd paid more attention at maths in school, but I stopped understanding it as soon as the alphabet got involved with x and flippin' y.

'Carry the six, cross out the two and make it a one, take away two—'

'Nineteen stone exactly.'

My surgeon had it quickly calculated. My eyelashes touched my eyebrows. I had purposely been avoiding the scales to remain unaware of this information. '*Nineteen stone?!* Christ on a tricycle! Oh thank God I am here. Please, please help me!' I begged him.

We discussed my weight gain, dieting history, my PCOS and all sorts of in-depth details. I loved how thorough he was. I told him I'd researched the bejaysus out of the whole thing and that I wanted to get a gastric band. But then he informed me that the gastric band procedure is not commonly performed any more as international results on a long-term basis are not proving to be good because patients are finding a way to 'eat around' the band. Janey mac. I couldn't believe it. Of course, because of my previous history of yo-yo dieting, it wouldn't be recommended for me. 'You're dead right. I bet I'd be one of those people who would have her cake and literally eat it too,' I thought.

'So what would be suitable for me, then?' I asked him. He suggested a gastric bypass. I had researched this in my wide-ranging studies, naturally. 'A gastric bypass?! But is that not for people who are so big they have to get firefighters to come and remove the side of their house, winch them out by a crane and take them in a reinforced ambulance to hospital?!' I wondered. Apparently not. I had watched a documentary called *The Fattest Man on Earth*. He weighed 75 stone and that's what he had done. Siobhan sidled in. 'Oh Jules, when are you going to get it in to your chubby little head? You have a BMI of 42. Hello? You are morbidly obese. Your waist is 44 inches. The circumference of each of your thighs measures 30 inches. That's what your waist measurement should be. You've got 50-inch hips for God's sake. This is life-saving surgery and you need it!' That was the one and only time that Siobhan made any sense.

I listened intently as my surgeon described in detail what a gastric bypass entailed. He then sent me off to think about it, saying he'd see me again in a month's time. I took to YouTube and watched the operation intently. Basically it involved key-hole surgery to divide the stomach into a large section and a much smaller section. The small part of the stomach is sewn together to make a pouch, which can hold only a cup or so of food. With such a small stomach, it means you feel full quickly and eat less. Once that's done, the surgeon disconnects the new small stomach pouch from the majority of the stomach and connects it to a part of the small intestine. The larger part of the stomach remains there and continues producing stomach acids as normal. In this new arrangement, food passes directly from the new small stomach into the intestine. This curbs the absorption of calories and nutrients and means that a highly nutritious diet must be consumed and that small portions of food must be eaten at regular intervals. This results in weight loss. That would mean I could get to my goal weight of ten stone. But hang on, it's irreversible surgery, meaning I could reach my goal, but I'd have to eat this way for the rest of my life. Woe. I lay back on my bed (yes, of course, eating) and pondered the long-term outcome.

'So this means that because I will have fewer opportunities to eat than with my current giant stretchy stomach, which can easily hold a big pizza no probs, with this gastric bypass I can only eat a ridiculously good diet of insanely healthy food in small portions and that will be for the rest of my life? What's not to love?! This is the tool I've been looking for! In fact, this is the chef, personal trainer, life coach and diet guru that I couldn't afford to have live with me 24/7, all rolled into one! Hallelujah! This is EXACTLY what I need.'

I am such an extremist. I'm all or nothing. So this new stomach system will keep me on the straight and narrow until my dying day when I'll be in a coffin for a normal-sized person, not one that they'll have to cut down an entire rainforest to make it big enough to fit me in! Great! I am all over this. Yes, please. Sign me up. 'Sold! To the fat lady in the front row.'

Happy as a pigeon outside a chipper at 4 a.m. on a Saturday morning, I continued my research. All seemed fine until I read this sentence: 'After a gastric bypass, due to the speed at which liquid now passes through the small stomach and directly enters the intestine, alcohol cannot be consumed.' My face blew back like when you open the oven door and it cremates you. Thank God I was lying down when I read it. Holy mother of all that is sacred. I'll never be able to drink booze again?!

This was obviously cataclysmic news. I wondered if they'd take my passport off me and revoke my Irish citizenship. No more of my beloved vodka. No more bonkers nights out. No more magic feeling *après* a few glasses of wine thinking, 'Ah lovely, that's taken the edge off. Jaysus, I feel mighty.' No more numb face and big happy head on me. No more being pissed and everything is just ten times funnier. No more losing my inhibitions and strutting my stuff on the dancefloor like I'm Beyoncé on a good hair day. Hang on, Jules, can you not think of any boons to this predicament? Okay. *long pause* No more waking up hangin' like a hanging basket, I suppose. No more blackouts. No more of the fear and feeling like I've maybe perhaps murdered several people like Jack the Ripper the previous night but have no recollection of it. No more waking up with my tongue as dry as a rice cake and a banging headache and feeling like the entire St Patrick's Day parade is marching in circles around my bed. No more reading the drunk texts I sent and then flinging the phone across the room in horror. No more seeing an empty wallet and a shedload of receipts for rounds of shots and bottles of Champagne lashed on the Visa card. Okay, maybe I can actually deal with this? Wait, hang on, that means when I do go out, I'm going to be Sober Sally. Oh God, no.

'What are ya havin', Jules?'

'Just a sparkling water, thanks, Tom.'

'You're not drinking?'

'No, I'm off the booze.'

'You are not! Will ya stop! C'mon, what are ya havin'?
Double vodka Red Bull, isn't it?'

'No really I'm not drinking because—'

'—you're on antibiotics?'

'No, I'm—'

'—you're preggers!'

'No! I'm not pregnant!'

'Ya are! Congrats! Who's the Da?!'

'Honestly, no, I'm just not drinking anym—'

'—Ah, you'll have the one! Go on! Just the one and
then we'll see after that. Sure you can leave the car
here and I'll bring you down to collect it tomorrow.
Even if I'm dyin' a death, I promise I'll bring ya down
to get it.'

'Honestly, Tom, I'm just not—'

'—Do you want a large one? And a drink to go with
it! Hahaha!'

'—Tom, I'm really not drinking, I—'

'—Jules, when I texted ya, I didn't say we were going out, I said we were going out out!'

'I know that but—'

'Barman! A double vodka Red Bull, a Jack and Coke, four Sambucas, two Jagerbombs and two pints of Bulmers, please! Cheers! Stick it on my credit card there, mister barman! Sure feck it! We'll worry about it tomorrow, eh Jules? Get that into ya Cynthia! Wooooo! I've had THE worst week at work! Let's get on the escape train and blow off some steam on the way to banterland! Choo! Choo! This is gonna be the best night EVER! Did you bring your passport with ya? Sure God only knows where we might wake up, wha'?!'

How in the name of Ginny Hendricks and tonic was I going to deal with that conversation every time I went out? And I am normally the one being Tom! I think in Ireland we don't like when the stone-cold soberers are on a night out for two reasons. No. 1: They are witnesses. As we all get baloobas and lose the run of ourselves, talk shite, make tits of ourselves and reveal all our true inner thoughts, the soberers are eye-witnesses to all of this and can remember all of it when we can't. And we don't like that because it feels like they have one up on us. We want everyone to be in the messy puddle of booze together. United we stand and legless we fall. No. 2: They make us feel guilty. Now there's a big difference between the civilised moderation of having a couple of drinks and enjoying them or a nice Shiraz with your steak dinner. I'm talking about getting on the beer bus to get elephants, like our infamous line from *Damo & Ivor*'s hit song: 'Everybody's drinkin' just to get drunk.' And so many of us go out to do just that and so we hate it when we meet a sober person and they give us that 'look' of disdain, the one that tells us we must look like Bambi on ice having just been shot with a tranquilliser dart and we spout absolute shite into their ear as we hang off their shoulder and the poor thing is just standing there having to listen to us waffle on incoherently while wanting to just face palm us out of the way and go home. Like that poor guy Jonathan who works in House bar on Leeson Street and every time I go in there, I make him hug me 'for at least ten seconds as that's how long you need for a decent hug'. Sorry, Jonathan. So even though we're langers, we can still see the aversion in the sober person's eyes and it makes us feel guilty for being such a drunken eejit. Why can't we do it in moderation and just stay in a nice happy drunk state for the entire night? Why do we have to get so lubricated that we become stupid, bedraggled, incompetent versions of ourselves? Answers on a postcard, please.

After a month I returned to my surgeon and told him about the research I'd conducted into gastric bypass and that I had decided it was the way to go for me. I was ready to commit for life as this was the intervention I needed. I couldn't cope with the thoughts of getting any bigger as I was already so unhappy and uncomfortable at this size. He told me the next port of call was a series of blood tests, an ECG monitor to check out my heart to see if it could withstand surgery, a visit to an endocrinologist to appraise my hormones and a psychological evaluation to ensure that I would be able to cope with this mentally. We discussed all the possible risks and complications that come with surgery, and there were many. And we talked about life post-surgery and how I would live with this smaller stomach. Alcohol came up in the conversation. 'I know, I know, I can't drink it ever again, but if it's one of the sacrifices I have to make, then I am willing to do it,' I assured him. 'You can still drink alcohol post-op – you'll just have a very low tolerance, as in one or two glasses of wine could get you drunk,' he informed me. 'So I can still drink?!' I exclaimed. 'Yes, but as I said, only a small amount, nothing like you've been drinking before.' 'Yeah, yeah, yeah, that's grand! I'm delighted! I love my nights out! Aw, this is turning out to be the best decision I ever made!' I said. 'Well, let's wait and see, there's a few more things we have to check first to ensure that you're a good candidate for surgery.' And flaming hoops they were too.

When my blood test results came back, all was grand except that I was deficient in vitamin D – very common for people in Ireland apparently, with our constant rain and clouds, and of course how could I not be deficient in it seeing as I had been practically wearing a nun's habit for so long that only my face and hands had seen a ray of sunshine in the past 15 years? So I was put on a course of vitamin D and sent off for six weeks. I loved how he was constantly monitoring me to make sure I wasn't looking for a quick fix. I'm sure people go in there saying, 'Well my daughter's getting married in six months and I need to lose six stone so here's my cheque book, let's make it happen!' But this ain't no quick fix, or cosmetic surgery, this is a medical intervention for the disease that is obesity.

My consultations continued for six months, which was great as my surgeon got to know me as a person and properly evaluate me and my intentions before he finally told me that he thought I was ready for surgery. I felt like jumping out of the extra-large chair he has for us big patients and kissing him on the forehead! 'Just one last question,' I said. This had been something I had avoided asking him for fear that it was going to crush my dream, but I had been working on positive visualisations with the law of attraction that I would have saved enough money to cover the cost of it. 'How much exactly is the surgery going to be?' I asked him. And I was told that because of my PCOS, it was covered on my health insurance. 'Exsqueeze me? What?! It's covered?!' I was not expecting that. You know that feeling when you buy a chocolate bar from a vending machine and then two bars fall out? Well multiply that by a zillion. I was ecstatic as I skipped out of the office and rang Dad to tell him the good news. 'Dad! I qualified for surgery and it's all covered on the VHI! Will you come car shopping with me?' And I went out with the money I had saved for surgery and treated myself to a sexy red BMW and thought, 'I am gonna look like a total ride when I'm a size 10 and driving around in this wearing a bikini!'

I hadn't told anyone but Mum and Dad that I had been considering weight-loss surgery for fear that if I didn't qualify, people would know how desperate I was to lose weight and had failed at yet another attempt to do something about it. The day I got my date for surgery was the day I finally had hope. It was scheduled for 1 November 2014. I was guaranteed to lose weight this time. I was also risking my life in the process, but I felt very confident with my surgeon because he had performed thousands of gastric bypass operations. I started a pre-op diet two weeks beforehand in order to shrink the size of my liver so it wouldn't get in the way, thus making the surgery easier to perform. I had planned to take a month off work to recover and since Andy had headed off to

Australia to chase the girl he'd fallen in love with, it was the perfect time for me to focus on myself and achieve the No. 1 thing that needed sorting out in my life.

Ten days before surgery I was called in to a meeting in RTÉ to talk about a project they wanted me to work on, but of course I had to tell them that I wasn't going to be around for the coming weeks as I was going under the knife. I also told them that I was going to take my camera with me and vlog the experience as nobody on YouTube had done it and I wished someone had. 'Well, if you're going to film it anyway, why not go the whole hog and make a TV documentary about it?' they asked. Why hadn't I thought of that?! 'Seriously? Could we do that?' I gasped. They thought it would be a great story to tell and could inspire a lot of people. 'My surgery is in ten days, we're gonna have to work fast.' And that we did. Ruth from *Damo & Ivor* came on as our producer and we enlisted Aoife Kelleher to direct it. I loved Aoife from the minute I met her and knew she was the right person to tell my story because she wouldn't make it sensationalist. I wanted it to be a classy documentary and Aoife was the right classy storyteller for the job.

I thought about what I'd want to see if I was watching the show myself and I knew the most important thing was to be 100% honest about what my body looked like and how I felt about it. So I said I'd like to go on camera in my underwear and show the viewers the reality of what 19 stone of obesity looks like and what my thoughts about it were. I still can't believe I did it; it was both terrifying and liberating in equal measure. I remember the sweat running down my back and praying that it wouldn't show up on camera. HD can be so cruel. I untied my robe and let it drop to the floor and I stood in front of the mirror, displaying my flab while the camera rolled. I talked about every square inch of my body and what I didn't like about it: the cellulite; the rolls of fat; my bloated pillow face that was so puffy I looked like I was constantly having a massive allergic reaction, like I'd been stung by a billion bees; my gigantic thighs that rubbed together; my chubby hands and fat fingers; my everything … I hated all of it. The only redeeming thing I could say was that I liked my face, but I felt it was lost in a puddle of fat. And I also mentioned that I was grateful for having a body in the first place. I was lucky to have arms and legs and not be disabled, I knew that, but I just wanted to be brutally honest about the way I felt about my excess weight. There was no point in lying. I knew that so many people watching would identify with me and think, 'that's how I feel when I look in the mirror', so I wanted to let viewers know that they weren't alone. I too hated myself.

When I did my main interview for the documentary I told Aoife beforehand that it wasn't going to be a big teary break-down-crying interview like you usually see on TV. I knew that because I wasn't emotional about it at all. I'm an emotional person, but I cry mostly at happy things. And I knew there wasn't a deep, dark traumatic event from my past that we'd discuss and I'd start bawling and say, 'After that I just started eating and couldn't stop.' Aoife asked if there was anyone in my family or friends who disagreed with me getting the surgery. I told her there wasn't but knew, as I'm a TV producer myself, that this would have been great as we could have interviewed them saying, 'I think she's making a big mistake here, this is too extreme,' and then interview them at the end crying and saying, 'I was wrong. This is the best decision she's ever made and I'm delighted for her that she's turned her life around.' That would be great telly. But I was surrounded only by people who thought that I was making a good decision and who completely supported me. But if there had been some knob jockey telling me not to do it, I would have disregarded their opinion anyway as everything in my being was telling me that this was going to be the best decision I would ever make.

I thought about what I'd have for my last death-row meal because post-op I would never be able to eat anything very greasy or sugary again. The reason I wouldn't be able to was that it could lead to 'dumping syndrome'. In layman's terms, if I ate something like that post-op, the fat and sugar would overwhelm my intestines so much that they would go into a panic and pretty much hit the emergency button and evacuate, so I'd feel really nauseous and get the scuthers. Charming. So I mentally penned a menu of my last supper and decided it would be a taste of all my favourite foods, which I'd eat in one epic day of sheer indulgence. On the bill of fare was: a big, fat, medium rare, juicy Shanahan's fillet steak with creamy mashed potatoes; macaroni and cheese sauce; prawn cocktail; pepperoni pizza; a full Irish fry-up with all the trimmings; a McDonald's quarter-pounder meal; Haagen-Dazs pralines and cream ice-cream; a big bowl of Coco Pops; copious amounts of chocolate bars; a bag of chipper chips drownded in vinegar; and a chicken fillet roll and a packet of Tayto cheese and onion crisps. Flippin' delish. And you know what's gas? In the end I decided not to have the death-row day. The more I thought about it, the more I realised how much I glorified food. I was worse than the boys in the orphanage in *Oliver Twist*. And I think making that decision to abstain from a planned day of gluttony was the beginning of me healing my relationship with food. The second step was admitting to myself that it wasn't just my hormones that were to blame for my weight. Yes, they made me prone to storing excess fat, but the reason I was fat was because I ate too much food and didn't exercise. It was entirely my fault. I was in this prison of fat because I had consciously committed the crime and handed myself this sentence. Nobody put that food in my mouth but me. Every unhealthy choice I made was my own doing. Every time I said 'Feck it' and shovelled something into my mouth it was my decision. I was responsible for my size, hormonal influence or not. I was fat because I had made myself fat.

I got further confirmation of this watching an episode of *Oprah* where she urgently summoned Dr Phil to fly to her house via her private jet, as ya do, where she was having dinner with 'the girls' and they needed help in solving a problem.

> Oprah: Dr Phil, we need you to tell us why we're fat.
>
> Dr Phil: You interrupted my dinner with my family and flew me hundreds of miles to ask me that?
>
> Oprah: Yes, it troubles us all deeply.
>
> Dr Phil: Hmm, I see. Well, here's the quick answer. I can probably make it home for dessert. You're fat because you want to be.
>
> The girls: We've been talking about it all weekend, as we can't figure it out ourselves. So we really need you to tell us.

Dr Phil: Oh so you want the honest answer?

The girls: Yes, we are ready for it.

Dr Phil: Okay, you're fat because you want to be.

Oprah: No really. You can tell us, we can take it.

Dr Phil: Oh, now I see. You want the whole truth ... Okay, you're fat because you want to be.

Dr Phil went on to explain that all of their choices in the past had caused them to gain weight. Nobody had forced them to make these choices regarding food and exercise; they made them because they wanted to. From the girls' perspective they had never chosen to be fat, but from Dr Phil's perspective the choices they had made in the past had clearly led to their present weight. They chose their actions and the resulting consequences. They wanted to be slim, but they made choices as though they wanted to be fat. So when presented with those daily decisions when thinking 'I'm hungry', they chose a doughnut over a salad. In those moments they didn't think, 'Do I want to be slim or fat?' No, they just thought 'Feed me' and then that good-tasting, fatty, sugary food that they ate months ago and gave them a few minutes' pleasure had the predictable consequence of making them fat now. How can you argue with that? It is completely true.

I wasn't nervous when the big day of surgery rolled around. Unfortunately the camera crew weren't allowed to tag along, so I took my own little camera along with me to vlog the experience. Never having been in hospital for anything before, I wasn't sure what to expect. The nurses were so lovely and kind. I donned the plus-size disposable knickers and gown they had laid out for me and was taken down to the operating theatre, only to have to return to remove my make-up as they would need to see the colour of my complexion under the anaesthetic, in case I was going pale. I had a full face of fake tan on too. Whoops. When I saw the theatre it was nothing like I had imagined. In my head it was huge and completely white. This one had stainless steel walls and looked like the inside of an industrial fridge. I hopped up on the operating table and met the lovely anaesthetist whose job it was to keep me sedated and, most importantly, alive for the next few hours. I had the banter with him and then had one overwhelming sudden moment of 'Oh holy crapola, what have you let yourself in for, Jules?!' when I spied several nurses unwrapping the metal surgical tools. There were loads of them and they were huge and I couldn't believe they were going to be inside me. After a few seconds of this disturbing thought, I shook my head to snap out of it and turned to the anaesthetist and said, 'Send me to the land of the unicorns. I'm ready, baby!' And with that I was in cloud cuckoo land for the next few hours as my insides were restructured. The gastric bypass was to my digestive system what the M50 motorway is to Dublin's traffic.

I woke up four hours later feeling incredible. Drenched in morphine, I was as high as a firefighter on a ladder attempting to put out a blaze in a marijuana factory. I was wheeled back to my room and greeted by my very relieved mum, who had been waiting patiently for my return. I had IV drips in my arms, a tube coming out of my nose that was attached to a bag of green gunge and a catheter stuck up my cha-cha. I was so spaced I didn't care what was hanging out of me. My hand repeatedly clicked what I called the 'Unicorn Button', which administered the morphine. For the following 24 hours, I was pain-free and smiling like Cheech and Chong. When I'd rinsed the bag of painkillers, the reality of the pain really set in. I felt like I'd been in one of those machines they have in a scrapyard for crushing cars. So I just kept repeating to myself, 'It will pass. It will pass.' I hadn't eaten for three days and you'd think at that stage I'd eat the backdoor buttered, but when they brought me some food, I was repulsed. I never, ever thought I'd be repelled by the sight of food, but when they wanted me to eat some puréed chicken, gravy and mash I had to force myself to eat a few spoonfuls. I had no feelings of hunger whatsoever. I told my vlog camera, 'Me and food are getting a divorce.' After three days in hospital, I returned home to Mum and Dad's house as I needed some minding. I thought I'd stay there for a few days, but it ended up being three weeks. I had five scars across my belly, ranging from half an inch to two inches in size. They were bigger than I had expected and looked so severe with the staples in them. As I peeled off the bandages for a peep, I knew I was going to be left with mingin' scars, but if that was the price I had to pay for a ticket to slimdom, then so be it.

Initially all of my food had to be puréed. I ate just baby food and soup for the first couple of weeks while my insides healed. It was easy enough as I had no feelings of hunger pangs like I used to beforehand. I injected myself daily with a needle filled with a drug to prevent me getting a blood clot, as this was one of the possible side-effects of surgery. The needle terrified me, but so did possible death by blood clot, so I just stuck it in my tummy every day to thin my blood and prevent such an atrocity. I was in a lot of pain for three full weeks, and then it started to get more bearable. Like a weaning toddler, I moved on to solid foods. My new diet was high in protein, loaded with vegetables, low in carbs and relatively the same size portions as a toddler's. As time went on I was able to eat more and more, with my maximum capacity being one cup.

I was eating a small-portion, highly nutritious meal every hour from morning to night. My jaw dropped when I stood up on the scales and I saw that I'd lost three stone in the first two months. Six weeks in, I started exercising. Before that, the only part of my body getting in shape was my eyebrows. Initially it was just walking. I got out and pounded the pavement for one hour every single day. I was puffing, panting and sweating like a pony after only five minutes, but I persisted because I wanted to get fit and knew I was going to have to work hard to burn off these pounds because it couldn't be done through diet alone if I wanted to get to my goal weight as fast as possible. I was literally going to have to work my ass off.

Did you ever wonder where the fat goes when you lose it? To hell, I'd like to imagine. So I looked it up to find out. As we know, fat is basically stored energy (funny that, considering when you're overweight you're knackered all the time). When you consume calories beyond what your body needs, you end up storing that extra energy in the form of triglycerides within the fat cells. When you successfully lose weight, your body converts the excess fat into usable energy for your muscles and other tissues through a series of complex metabolic processes. This causes your fat cells to shrink. If someone was to lose 10 kg of fat (triglyceride), 8.4 kg is exhaled as $CO_2$ while the remaining 1.6 kg is lost as water in urine, faeces, sweat, tears and other bodily fluids. So when fat is lost, it is mostly exhaled as carbon dioxide, with the remainder being excreted as water. So that means that the lungs are the primary excretory organ for fat! Well if I'd read that a few years ago, I probably would have started the hyperventilating diet and no doubt fainted within a few minutes.

**If you want to lose weight, the next two paragraphs need your particular attention.**

After the initial rapid weight loss, things then slowed down as my body tried to adjust to the new regime. Thinking it was in a famine-type state, after 12 weeks the losses began to plateau and there were weeks when I didn't lose a pound. Thankfully, I had been warned that this would happen. As part of the documentary, I met nutritionist Elsa Jones, who showed me a football and told me that was the size an average person's stomach could stretch to when full of food. Then she showed me a tennis ball and explained that this was my new capacity – for life. We discussed all things nutrition and how I was going to eat for the rest of my life and then Elsa broached the topic of uncovering the emotional reason behind why I had eaten the way I did. I told her I had looked into it and couldn't find an incident or issue from the past that could have caused me to eat for comfort or to fill a void. Elsa thought it interesting that I didn't consider myself to be an emotional eater because I had automatically thought that I should be looking for something negative, like eating if you're upset, sad, tired or frustrated. Then she explained that 'most of us actually do our eating in relation to positive emotions and eat when we want to seek pleasure, to reward ourselves, for example.' 'Eureka! Oh my God! That's me! That's my thing! I eat to reward myself!'

Elsa had hit the nail on the head. It resonated perfectly with me. This is the revelation I had spent years searching for! I ate to reward myself for my achievements. I'd tell myself I was great and deserved to have the croissant with the cup of coffee because I'd earned it for doing a good day's work or just being a good all-round person – let's be honest, it didn't take much for me to sell it to myself as to why I deserved a treat. I could think of a valid reason in a nanosecond. 'It's Friday! Feck it!' But why was I rewarding myself with food in the form of treats when I am not a dog?

Such a lightbulb went off that day with the discovery of the original root cause of my weight gain. I came home that evening and thought about it some more. I had pinpointed Ios as the place it all began, but now I realised that what Ios was really all about was me rewarding myself with a holiday of indulgence. I ate and drank myself stupid. I didn't do a tap of work. I was completely irresponsible and lived beyond my means and had a fab time doing it. I was the mayoress of Treat City. Population: Me. But that's not the reality of life. I'm not a bleedin' Kardashian. But treating myself felt good and that's why I continued to do it afterwards, without realising it was coming with catastrophic consequences. I also realised that even after I'd had the gastric bypass, I was STILL doing it. I was eating low-fat crisps alongside my super-healthy diet.

So even with the intervention of radical surgery, I discovered that if you don't heal your head, you're fecked. I threw all the crisps in the bin and I set about creating a new habit for the following 21 days, as that's the length of time it takes to reprogramme your mind with a new habit of thinking. Every single time I thought about rewarding myself or I had an option to reward myself with food, I said a very loud 'NO!' in my head and shut the press. I used my Reiki training to clear the energy and as I did this, I said the mantra, 'I love and approve of myself. I am in control. I create my own security. I am safe.' This really empowered me and after 21 days of practising it, it became a new habit and I stopped rewarding myself with treats and saw food in a whole new light: it was just fuel. I had healed my emotional eating and with my head healed, my body could now fall into line and be slim because it didn't need to reflect back to me what I needed to sort out emotionally. The weight could now finally come off and, most importantly, stay off. So the biggest revelation that I have uncovered on my journey and analysis of weight loss is that it is essential to heal the emotional cause behind your weight gain, otherwise you will continue the cycle of diet and doom, losing weight and putting it back on, because the main crux of the problem hasn't been fixed. You may already know what your emotional cause is or you may not, but I suggest to everyone I discuss this with to visit a therapist and work it out and release it, then your body can breathe a sigh of relief and drop the pounds forever. My problem was an addiction to treating myself with food. I finally managed to overcome that addiction once I'd figured out the original root cause. The comfort eating was an after-effect, but I believe uncovering and healing the emotional cause is the key to it all.

Here are some wise words that explain addiction simply.

> If you require a certain result in order to
> be happy, you have an addiction. If you
> simply desire a certain result, you have
> a preference. If you have no preference
> whatsoever, you have acceptance. You
> have achieved mastery.

> Neale Donald Walsh (author)

And these are the differences.

> The Addict: I couldn't give a flying fuck about my diet. If I don't have this bar of chocolate right now, I will actually die! I mean I will keel over and literally die!

> The Desirer: I'd love to eat that bar of chocolate but instead of telling myself 'I CAN'T eat it because I'm on a diet,' I choose to say 'I DON'T eat chocolate because I am empowered and engaged in a healthy eating lifestyle where I only eat foods that nourish my body.'

> The Master: Does the chocolate bar even exist?

> The Addict: Not any more! I just ate it! Sorry!

One of the scariest experiences post-op was looking at my hairbrush and seeing it crammed with hair after just one brush. My hair fell out at an alarming rate and it was terrifying. It didn't come out in clumps, but it would just be all over my hands as I washed it and the hairbrush would fill up with just one blow-dry. I had been warned it was a very common side-effect as the hormones rebalanced in the body, but I had brushed it off and thought, 'I'm fab. It won't happen to me.' But oh yes it did.

Hair loss happens to a lot of women post-pregnancy and it can also happen as a result of stress and lots of other reasons. My hair was long and thick and when it started to disappear, I felt like my mojo was dissipating, like Samson with a blade-one. I'm a Leo and my mane is important to me. It holds a lot of my self-confidence. In total about half, maybe more, of my hair fell out. It was heartbreaking as I brushed the thin strands that had managed to hang on. It'll take me a good three years to grow it all back and because my baldy barnet was really getting me down, I decided to do something about it. I visited a salon to get hair extensions. I thought I was getting them for beauty reasons, so I could see luscious locks in the mirror and have the wondrous feeling of having hair to run my fingers through again, but it turned out to be even more of an experience because I found myself getting emotional as I walked out the door with my new voluminous, long locks swishing in the wind like I was in a shampoo ad. I hadn't expected that. I knew the hair loss was upsetting me, but it wasn't until I suddenly had hair back that I realised how much. I talked about hair loss on my Snapchat one day and I was inundated with messages back from women telling me about theirs. I had no idea that so many women were affected by it. Thankfully, the hair extensions gave me back a great sense of power and confidence. I had never known that I had put such a value on my hair. It's true when they say you don't know what you've got until it's gone, for example: toilet paper.

I don't think anything or anyone could have prepared me for the mind-fuck of losing so much weight so fast. In five months I had rapidly shrunk from 19 stone and a size 22, down through all the clothes sizes to a size 14 and weighing 13 stone. While my body had accelerated towards my goal weight, my head had not. I got a fright every time I saw a photo of myself, literally recoiling when I saw a picture as I'd be so startled that I only had one chin. The same with catching a glimpse of myself in a mirror or window reflection. It was so shocking that it took a full year from the surgery date for my mind to catch up and register that I wasn't fat any more. *You are slim, Jules. You are actually slim.* 'Is this a dream?' I'd ask myself. Nope, this is your new life. All of my family and friends were thrilled for me and my transformation and endlessly commented on how great I looked, which is something I never tired of hearing. Mum bawled her eyes out when she saw me in a tight-fitting Jessica Rabbit-type dress. She was just so happy for me. In 2015, six months after surgery, I climbed a mountain with Andy as part of a challenge set out by personal trainer Karl Henry, with whom we filmed my documentary. Now it wasn't Everest, but it was a mountain that I certainly couldn't have even attempted a few months previously. When I was climbing down through the rocks, even though I was now so much lighter, I still had a tremendous fear that if I hopped from one rock to another my knees would give way and break under the heavy load I thought I was still carrying. Throughout this time, which now feels like a blur as everything happened so quickly, Siobhan was on a hiatus, you'll be glad to hear. I think she was so in shock that I was finally overpowering her that she was literally speechless, standing there frozen like a statue, and she didn't speak for months, apart from the odd bit of drivel, but I quickly shut her up.

While my mind was like a gigantic jigsaw trying to put itself together, my body was flourishing and working in hormonal harmony for the first time ever. Due to my new healthy eating plan, which was very low on sugar, my hormones regulated and I began getting a monthly period just like a normal woman. I had no PMT or bloating either, which I again put down to the low sugar intake as I believe sugar and hormones are mortal enemies. Now every 30 days lovely Aunt Flo pays a visit and she is a dream house guest, I'm delighted to report. So with my tomato soup back on the boil, I felt like I'd got my femininity back and because of my rediscovered womanhood, I started to enjoy clothes shopping again. The last time I'd worn anything that was in fashion was in the 1990s, so I had to find out what my 'style' was because I hadn't had one apart from my all-black 'nun chic' ensembles. I had to learn to switch off my blinkers, which had been trained for so long to only spy black, flowy clothes on the racks. I found myself bringing numerous different sizes into the changing rooms and thinking, 'I won't get into the 14', but then slipping into the size 12 and dancing around the cubicle like a lunatic and posing like I was Naomi Campbell on the runway. With this new-found confidence, I couldn't stop taking selfies and each time I posted a photo on my Facebook page, my friends left a flurry of comments about how great I looked. Nobody knew at this stage how much weight I'd lost or how I had done it. I decided to keep it all a secret until it came time to launch my documentary, *Nine Stone Lighter*.

On the final day of filming in August, I faced the last challenge that had been set for me by Karl Henry, which was to do a triathlon. When he'd revealed the task to me, on camera, two months previously, my eyes had popped and I'd blurted out, 'What's a triathlon?!', because I hadn't a notion. Of course I'd heard the word, but with as much interest in the world of fitness as a stoned koala, I had no clue as to what it entailed. He told me I was going to swim 250 m in the sea, cycle 20 km and run 5 km. My first thought was not the endurance it would take to complete the task, it was that I would have to wear a wetsuit. I instantly thought, 'I'm gonna look like a walrus', until I remembered that I wasn't big anymore and they would have one to fit me. Again, my mind and old thought patterns were still trying to catch up with my new slim body. Thankfully, the lovely Andy agreed to do the triathlon with me, to give me the moral support I needed. We started training and after the first bike ride the seat was so sore I felt like I'd been shagged lubeless by the Jolly Green Giant, and so did Andy. I got us some gel seat-covers to ease the crotch pain and that helped a lot. We ran, we swam, we cycled. I moaned and moaned and Andy gave me constant words of encouragement, a literal slap on the arse and also reminded me that this was going to be filmed, so there was no backing out. Tough shit.

We called over to our mate Gav, who had done loads of endurance runs and iron mans, to get some advice. After he told me about the endorphin rush of happiness and emotion I'd experience crossing the finish-line, I started to get excited. I had no clue whether I'd trained enough for the event or whether I'd be able to complete it. Gav recommended 'a big bowl of pasta the night before and a big bowl of porridge on the day to get the carbs in'. 'Hang on, Gav, I can't eat any of that! Jaysus, how am I going to fuel my body to get through this?' I panicked. 'What about the energy drinks? Could you have those?' he asked. I didn't know. I had avoided anything overly sugary after I had experienced the dreaded dumping syndrome once a few months previously. I had scoffed a cupcake covered in sugary icing and within minutes I felt sick and was running to the jacks. What if I had an energy drink mid-triathlon and was filmed cycling off-track into a bush, screaming and begging someone to please bring me some toilet paper or even some feckin' dock leaves?! Oh God, please don't let that happen.

On the day of the triathlon I trembled with nerves. I had managed to get into my wetsuit with ease; in fact, I was wearing a size small. We lined up at the starting point on Greystones beach. The horn blew and 200 of us ran full pelt into the freezing cold sea. This was my first time in the sea in 15 years. I swallowed a big mouthful of water, gagged and threw it up but kept on going. Andy powered along beside me and kept shouting, 'You can do it.' I was gasping for breath by the time we reached the shoreline again and somehow managed to drag myself back to the base camp to begin the struggle of peeling off the wetsuit, a similar experience to Colin Farrell taking off a johnnie, I imagine, but I was so weak I didn't have the strength to throw my leg over my bike. With zero energy, I began to shake. 'Feck it,' I thought as I grabbed the energy drink I'd brought in case of such a predicament and I horsed it into me, praying I wouldn't get an attack of bum gravy mid-cycle. I hadn't had that much sugar in my system for ten months and I felt like Stephen Roche after a Galtee cheese sandwich for the cycling part. We sailed through it, and then it was on to the 5 km run. If Andy wasn't there with me, I don't know how I would have got through it.

When the finish-line and the crowds came in sight, it was their cheering that got me to take the last steps over the line. I was absolutely delirious with the exhaustion and within minutes collapsed on the ground like a new-born lamb. 'Where's the endorphin rush and the overwhelming emotion that everyone told me I'd get?' I wondered. I think my sugar levels had crashed so low that I had gone Star Trekkin' across the universe. The paramedics checked me over and told me I'd live. I guzzled some more energy drink and that brought me round. Everyone told me it was an incredible achievement and asked if I'd do it again, to which I replied, 'Not in a million feckin' years.' Andy was buzzing like a madman and asking how he could sign up for the next one. 'I'm just gonna stick to the gym, Ted,' I told him.

On that day I weighed ten stone nine pounds. I was just over half a stone away from my goal weight, but it felt like I was already there. After the triathlon, and probably the nicest shower I've ever had in my life, I disrobed for the cameras once more, to show my new body. Surprisingly, it was just as terrifying as the first time I did it, even though I was now pretty much half the size I was before, yet twice the woman I used to be. My waist was now a healthy 30 inches – the original size of my thigh! My body looked great, but I was still complaining. Thankfully, I hadn't suffered much excess skin and I put this down to all the exercise I did. I just had a bit of saggy skin on my inner thighs, my lower belly, arms and bum. I showed the camera how I pulled back the skin on my thighs and wondered, 'Is this what I'd look like with a thigh lift?' I wanted to be brutally honest about the thoughts I was having and not stand there and say, 'Everything is perfect now that I'm slim', because the truth was I was still looking for things to fix. I had been wondering if I should get a boob job because I'd lost so much shape in the upper part of my Brad Pitts since they'd deflated from an E-cup to a B-cup. But then I realised that if I did that, then I'd move on to wanting to correct something else. I asked the camera, 'Will I ever be happy with my body? ... Will any woman ever be happy with her body?' Now, thanks to Dante the child genius, I knew that perfection did not exist. My next project was to love my body and embrace the fact that it was 'good enough'.

Watching the editing of *Nine Stone Lighter* come together was surreal. In 50 minutes, I go from fat to slim. We also filmed an internal scan of my womb, during which I discovered that my PCOS was all but 'cured'. The cysts on my ovaries were gone, my periods were regular and my hormones completely balanced. This means that when I want to start a family, it is now a possibility. It was a touching moment to know that my eggs weren't being stupid eejits anymore and had finally discovered the entrance to Copper Face Jacks. A couple of weeks after filming ended, I stepped on the scales and saw ten stone staring back at me. I had hit my goal. It felt AAAMAZING! I actually feckin' did it and everyone was thrilled for me.

Along the journey the only person who wasn't sure if I would be able to do it was an endocrinologist, Professor Donal O'Shea, who we had interviewed as part of the documentary. I really enjoyed our chat that day. He's a lovely man and a leading expert on obesity who championed bariatric surgery being put back on the public health system, which is absolutely fantastic for anyone who needs this intervention but can't afford to have it done privately or on health insurance. Our very interesting hour-long conversation that day could have been an entire documentary in itself. However, in *Nine Stone Lighter* the only part that made it into the edit was this small segment of our chat.

'Do you have a target weight?'

'Eleven stone was my original goal, but I've changed it in the past few months to ten and a half. So I have another three to go.'

'If I told you that you were very unlikely to achieve that and you were likely to stop at about 11 or 11 and a half stone based on all the international evidence, how would you feel about that?'

'Part of me wants to say, "Yeah, I would be okay with that," but then realistically, deep down, if I'm very honest, I wouldn't.'

'I fear from what I've heard from you so far, you've described yourself as all or nothing and so far it's all the "all" bit. Have you planned for failure in the post-gastric bypass you?'

'Planning around failure would be the opposite of my personality. So, em, I haven't thought about any of those sort of things, of going "What if I don't get to my goal?" Because I think nearly in my head I'm already there. So I'm going for that goal.'

'You will then have a new weight to defend and work hard to keep steady. I think that'll be closer to 12 stone. You're hoping it's going to be closer to 11?'

'Ten. Ten and a half.'

'Ten and a half? You know, we'll see. But either way the challenge in the weight management area is out at 18 months and two years, stopping the regain and a lot of

the surgeries now being done in the US are
second surgeries for people because the
regain has been a big problem.'

Second surgeries? Do you see what I mean now about
the healing your head bit? I could have been one of
those. I might have lost loads of weight and then
regained it if I had kept rewarding myself with food
even though I'd had a gastric bypass. When *Nine Stone
Lighter* aired, lots of people sent messages saying, 'Ha!
You showed yer man who said you couldn't get to ten
stone! Well done!' But by the end of that conversation,
which wasn't included in the documentary, I think
Professor O'Shea knew that I would. He didn't know
me from Adam when he met me, so he didn't realise
at first that he was talking to someone who had healed
her head and therefore wasn't going to fall into the
category of one of those international statistics.

So with the airing of *Nine Stone Lighter* came the
press junket and because everyone loves a weight-loss
story, I was everywhere. I donned my size 22 jeans
for a photoshoot and showed how they were now
swimming on me. All the papers and magazines picked
up the story and I was morto going into the newsagent
to buy the *Daily Mail* when I saw a big photo of
myself on the cover. I folded the paper in half and
put it on the counter in case the clerk thought I was a
vain bitch. My biggest interview was when I went on

*The Late Late Show*, to have a chat with Ryan Tubridy. Of course, my first thought was, 'What'll I wear?!' I chose a tight-fitting red dress that looked like one you'd see in a Special K ad. I've been in the RTÉ studios a billion times in the past 20 years since I first went there for my school work experience aged 16. It's a second home, so I wasn't nervous at all about going out live to half a million people around Ireland, all watching on their sofas while drinking wine and eating crisps. Ryan Tubridy was so nice to me that I wasn't afraid he was going to throw me any clanger questions; he'd had a sneak preview of the documentary and really liked it. And even if he had caught me off-guard, I would have answered as best I could because I was talking about my specialist subject: me.

My main goal that night was to not snot myself walking down the steps in my red heels as I was still getting used to wearing them, having been in nothing but flats for so long. Once I didn't tumble down and show the nation my Bridget Jones sausage-casing knickers (yes, I was still wearing them, as a girl can't be sucked in enough, no matter what size she is!), everything else was going to be a win. So after I ducked down behind the life-size cardboard cut-out they had of me as DJ Deirdre and was introduced, I popped up, did a cheeky wiggle and managed to make it down the three steps. Phew! As soon as I sat on the sofa, the adrenaline started pumping and my mouth went so dry I felt like I'd just eaten a bag of sawdust. That was all I could think of as I somehow managed to do the interview. When I headed back to the green room, I was convinced my Sahara mouth must have been so evident, everyone must have thought I was a basket-case of nerves when I wasn't, it was just a saliva malfunction! But my best mate Donna assured me that I sounded great and it wasn't noticeable at all. 'Oh thank God! Here, give us a vodka to soak up the sawdust, thanks, Teddy!' was my reply.

The morning after my appearance on *The Late Late Show*, hangin' like a loose tooth, I hauled my ass to the gym to sweat out the vodka and there I was approached by Matt Keatley, one of the personal trainers, who told me that he'd seen me on TV the night before and had recognised me from the gym. He had no idea that I had been on such a mammoth weight-loss journey. We chatted about all things nutrition and fitness and also discovered that we were both on the same island of Ios that epic summer back in 1998. I had been thinking about getting a personal trainer, because at this stage I was finding the gym so boring and monotonous, just doing cardio all the time. After meeting Matt, I knew he was the man for the job. Little did I know on that day that he would have as much of an impact on my life as the surgery. What a difference having a personal trainer makes. In fact, I think it's essential if you want to get fit. The first obstacle I used to throw up was the cost of it. You're talking around 30 quid for a one-hour session, yet I don't bat an eyelid paying the same for a blow-dry, a round of drinks, getting my nails done, a new top. I spend even larger amounts of money on things like facials, massages, dinners out, I mean easily 100 quid on a flippin' hangover! I decided the 30 quid was a long-lasting investment in my body, because my body will be around a lot longer than that expensive handbag I simply had to have. I like to think of my PT sessions as a training class because every time I train with Matt, I'm learning how to work out properly. I'm discovering how to use the machines in the gym with good form and technique and, most importantly, Matt's encouraging me, motivating me and pushing me to do the best I can.

When I was in the gym by myself, because Siobhan hates exercise, she would just wail, 'Juuuules, this treadmilling is sooooo boring. We're just staring at a wall. You've already done 20 minutes on it! Is that not enough to appease the guilt? *sigh* How about we go to the café downstairs and get a nice little Al Pacino? Sure you've earned it now. And by the way, did I mention how your face is majorly sweaty? Hashtag beetroot. You look horrif. What if we bump into someone we know and they see the absolute state of you? Why couldn't you have just listened to me this morning and stayed in bed? We'd be all relaxed and cosy now if you'd just done as I said. You've done more than enough. I bet you'll be at your goal weight when you get on the scales tomorrow! You're way better off to just leave now. C'mon Jules, let's go, this is sooooo boring!' And I would have to scream back at her, 'SIOBHAN! You know this is not sweat pouring down my face and chest? It's vodka! Vodka is oozing from my pores! And whose fault is that? Yes, that's right, it's yours! If I was to lick my top lip right now, I'd be half cut! Now shut up, you stupid bitch!' But Siobhan wouldn't shut up. She'd continue nagging in my ear and soon enough I'd give in to her, hit the stop button and head to the changing rooms.

When I teamed up with Matt, I had someone who was actually on my side, not like Siobhan the mega-bitch. Matt asked what I wanted to achieve and I told him that, as I was now at my goal weight, I wanted to tone up my body and get some definition because I had a bit of saggy skin on my tummy, arms, inner thighs and my arse looked like I was on the beach wearing flesh-coloured bikini bottoms filled with sand. So he designed a training programme that was suitable for my body, ability and my goals. He had me lifting weights, doing resistance, going on all the machines I was too scared to touch and even going down into the heavy weights section that's full of grunting males making themselves into muscle beasts, which myself and the girls refer to as 'The Lions' Den'. Once I was with my personal trainer I found a confidence in the gym I never had before. It was always an overwhelming environment, but now that I had a guide, it became a place I could actually really enjoy.

Let the gainz begin! Within six weeks of starting training, I started to notice a huge difference in my body. I was lifting heavy weights and my arms were getting smaller in size yet revealing definition. I used to think lifting weights would turn me into a big bodybuilder and I'd look like a human croissant, but no, us girls don't have enough testosterone to do that, apparently. My body shape started changing and I loved it. Toned feckin' arms! Never thought I'd see the day! It makes such a difference in clothes, especially dresses, and when you see a photo of yourself on a night out and your arms don't look like big rolling pins hanging out of your shoulders, it feels fantastic, and then there's no need to crop the chunky arm out of the picture to make it your new profiler! I can't get over the difference between feeling fit and feeling fit and strong. It is incredibly empowering. I had the strength of a dead sparrow when I first started with Matt. I struggled to lift 4 kg dumbbells six months ago and now I've worked my way up to 12 kg ones. I've done so many squats I've got the tightest bottle of Bass in Dublin. With this proper training came the endorphin rush that up until now I had thought was purely a myth, or perhaps a marketing ploy that some gym manager had invented to encourage people to go to the gym but as it didn't exist, people would keep going to chase this coveted state of fitness nirvana. But as it turns out, it is true, and the wondrous endorphin rush is just as extraordinary as they say it is. How would I describe it? Well, imagine a majestic, beautiful unicorn brought out a range of vibrators enchanted with unicorn magic and then gave you one for free. Like that.

So now that I know what I'm doing in the gym I leave after my one-hour workout absolutely buzzing on a major high, yes with aching muscles, and sometimes my legs are so sore that I have to lower myself down on the toilet so slowly I'm like a 90-year-old granny crippled with arthritis, but that's when I know I've made progress and that my body shape is changing for the better as I get my tone on. The bottom line is, you don't get the ass you want by sitting on it. I was happy when I got to my goal weight, I had a body that looked good in clothes. Now, thanks to training effectively, I have a body that looks good nekked! I just need a feckin' boyfriend to show it to! And before you suggest it, no, there are no rides down in 'The Lions' Den'. Believe me, I've checked!

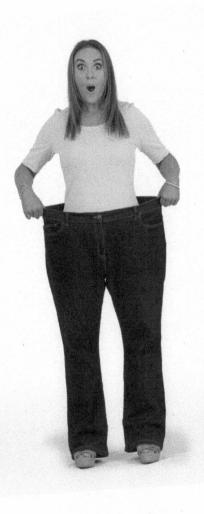

# 8

# The Ride & Prejudice

'*I* was happy for yer one from *Damo & Ivor* losing the weight until I heard she did it by surgery. The cheating fuck.'

That was the only negative message online when my documentary aired. I made a Facebook page to promote *Nine Stone Lighter* and the night it was shown on telly, the page was flooded with messages, way more than I had ever even expected. I was so surprised by the emotion people felt watching it. That is something I had not anticipated. There were so many people telling me that they were crying watching me as I stood at 19 stone in my underwear, describing all the things I hated about my body. They were crying because they felt the same about their bodies and thought they were the only ones who had such terrible thoughts about their rolls of flab. They were also bawling when Andy and I crossed the finish-line of the triathlon, and in floods when I discovered that my PCOS had all but disappeared and I could now have a baby. It was mad for me to realise that I used to be that girl who cried watching the weight-loss documentaries and now I was the subject of one and making other people weep.

So have all my insecurities disappeared now that I've lost the weight? Nope. Yes, they've dramatically diminished, but I believe insecurity is etched in our DNA and there ain't nothing we can do about it, apart from a lifelong task of trying to keep them to a minimum. Sure even the supermodels of this world have their qualms. Wouldn't it be wonderful if, in everyday life, we could all remember that everyone, no matter what they look like, is insecure? We are all just as insecure as each other. Every single one of us, all day, every day, insecure as fuck. I have received countless messages from lovely people telling me that I'm an inspiration and I am so glad I shared my journey to give people hope and show them that it can be done. So what did I do when I read that one negative message on Twitter? Well I could have gotten angry and tweeted back, 'Listen here, wagon features, I'll have you know that ...' But the moment you defend yourself, you start the war. So instead I chose to laugh and immediately asked myself, 'Okay, mirrors! This is not about the girl who wrote that message. This is about ME. What is this bringing up for clearing?' And I realised that she was reflecting back to me the issues I have with people who see weight-loss surgery as an 'easy option' or a way of losing weight by 'cheating' because they believe it should 'only be done by hard work through diet and exercise'.

So I asked myself, 'Do you believe that surgery is cheating?' and I knew straightaway that the answer was a big, fat no. If you have a heart attack and get triple-bypass surgery to stay alive, is that cheating? She was reflecting back the opposite to me, which can often happen with the mirrors. Having been through it all, I can tell you fo' shizzle that having weight-loss surgery is actually the most difficult way of all to lose weight. First off, you have to risk your life with the anaesthetic and the surgery itself and then survive any potential complications.

'How did she die?'

'Trying to make herself slim.'

'Jaysus. The poor fucker.'

'I know.'

Then you have to go through the agonising pain of recovery. Then you have to adjust overnight to a radical new way of eating and stick to it for the rest of your life – for example, I can't eat and drink at the same time, I have to choose one or the other. I'm used to it now in everyday life, but it's a real pisser on nights out. So I'm having a few glasses of vino with the girls and I think, 'I'd love a few peanuts to nibble on'. I have to put down the wine glass, wait ten minutes, eat the peanuts, wait 30 minutes, then pick up the wine glass again. Needless to say, that's why I don't eat many peanuts. But this is just one of the sacrifices I've had to make in order to have the intervention I so badly needed. On top of all that goes with surgery and adapting to a new way of eating and drinking, I still had to dedicate myself to a supremely healthy diet and exercise like a lunatic in order to shed the weight. I sweated like a human Niagara Falls to burn up that poundage. So I can categorically state that it is NOT an easy option to choose. It is, I believe, the hardest. That's why it's not just some form of cosmetic surgery. 'Oh yah, I just popped in for a gastric bypass on my lunch break and the following day I woke up skinny. Easy peasy! It's *fah*-bulous, dahling!' It's a medical intervention to cure the disease that is obesity. Having said all that, it is the best decision I ever made in my life and I would do it all again in a heartbeat! Fact.

So with my face all over the telly and in the press, of course people started to recognise me when I was out and about. I've watched Andy go through it for years, obviously on a much bigger scale than me, and I love it when people approach me to congratulate me on my weight loss. I mostly get recognised in the supermarket, for some reason, and it's always by women. Some of them literally root through my trolley to see what I'm buying as the biggest question I get asked is, 'What do you eat on a daily basis? Tell me, please!' The only thing they'll find in my trolley is healthy shite and at the weekends, a bottle of vodka. I put a phenomenal amount of dedication into my diet and meal-prep all my food in bulk because it makes life so easy. It means I only have to cook twice a week and then I bang it all into lunch-boxes and into the fridge and then grab and go, with the additional score of only having to do the washing-up twice a week too. Winning at life! From six months post-op, my ability to eat larger portions increased. I suppose you could say my capacity now is what should be a 'normal' healthy portion size, but it still looks relatively small because everyone eats gigantic amounts these days due to the supersize lifestyle we've become accustomed to over the years compared to how people ate back in the 1970s and before. I'm all about the clean eating twenty-four-sev. Lots of vegetables, protein, healthy fats and slow-release energy carbs. There's a full meal planner and recipes on my website (www.julescoll.com), showing how and what I eat.

I have to say my inner Irish leprechaun is delirah that I can still go out on the lasharoo. I just make sure I eat beforehand and my tipple of choice is vodka and soda water with a slice and a squeeze of fresh lime as that's the lowest sugar option and gives me the least hangover. If I drink wine, by comparison, it's so sugary I'll wake up feeling like something Shane McGowan just coughed up. I switched my crazy caffeine coffee and tea habit from five-plus cups a day to one, and I drink decaf the rest of the time and now I sleep like a dead man. I've become a big fan of matcha green tea too. I pop more pills than an entire nightclub in Ibiza with all the multivitamins and supplements I take. And I knock back a daily shot of apple cider vinegar and super-greens powder mixed with water. Absolute vomicide. It tastes like snogging a gremlin, but I just horse it into me for the health benefits.

I also live a fragrance-free life after learning that the chemical fragrances in perfume, aftershave, deodorants, scented candles, air-fresheners, detergents, fabric softeners, etc., all affect our central nervous system and have been shown to cause anxiety, panic attacks, headaches, migraines and disrupt our hormones. I rid my life of fragrances and noticed a huge difference in my mental clarity because I wasn't going around in a cloud of chemical fragrances anymore. I now use natural products and essential oils instead of perfume. So if you've ever wondered what I smell like, just imagine a woodland fairy that's rolled around in the rose bushes and bluebells of a secret garden.

Now that I have healed my emotional relationship with food, I can finally see food as fuel and nourishment for my body, which means I don't need to experience the feeling of needing 'treats'. I don't treat myself like a good dog because I now feel like a ride. It's just not on my radar these days because those things don't do it for me anymore. Now that I have empowered the word CHOICES in my life, I get a bigger reward from choosing to say no to any temptation as I know that being slim and healthy is better than any food I could ever eat and that buying clothes in a size 10 and fitting into them is the additional treat to every healthy choice I make. I now realise that eating junk food isn't a reward, it's a punishment. Healing the emotional reasons behind my weight gain has enabled me to become empowered to the point where I am, finally, in control of what I eat. I have often wondered what would have happened if I'd found out the emotional reason behind why I ate before I had surgery. Could I have healed it and then lost the weight without having a gastric bypass? I'll never know. But I do believe trying to lose weight without addressing the underlying emotional issue is like trying to drive a car with the handbrake on. I do get the odd hormonal craving for my ex-boyfriend chocolate, but when that happens I just have two squares of 85% dark chocolate. The cocoa is so much more concentrated than a milk chocolate bar, so it gives me a total chocolate fix in a very small amount. I used to hate dark chocolate but I have learned to love it. This Christmas, while pissed, I ate a Ferrero Rocher and my face contorted like Sloth from *The Goonies* because it was so sweet and sugary. I couldn't believe it. My tastebuds have obviously changed since I banished sugar from my diet and I don't miss it because sugar is the devil.

To avoid the dreaded dumping syndrome, I steered clear of any sugary or greasy foods. Thankfully, the absence of sugar in my body meant my hormones reset like pressing Ctrl, Alt, Delete on a computer. As Matt and I talk endlessly about nutrition during our PT sessions, one of our favourite subjects was the shit-stirrer that is sugar. He showed me how to read a food label to work out how many teaspoons of sugar a product contains. I became obsessed with plucking items off the shelf in the supermarket and calculating their sugar content and my gob would be hanging open in shock looking at most of them. I then discovered through Matt that excess sugar consumed is converted to fat by the body and stored. The average Irish person consumes 24 teaspoons of sugar a day – that's four times the daily allowance recommended by the World Health Organization. When I learned that, I was astonished. We are sugar junkies, so no wonder we're on course to becoming the fattest nation in Europe by 2030!

The ability to read a food label was such a huge eye-opener for me that I felt compelled to share it with more people, to give them the ability to know what was in their food and drinks and thereby make an informed choice, especially for parents feeding their children. I was close to tears one day in the supermarket reading the sugar content in yogurts packaged in branding aimed at kids and in 'light' yogurts targeted at people trying to lose weight. The shocking truth was that both brands each had three or four teaspoons of sugar in them. In order to spread awareness, Matt and I made two videos about the wiles of sugar in processed food and drinks and I posted them on Facebook. They instantly went viral and set the newsfeed ablaze. I felt very proud of those videos and the work we put into them to help people realise that sugar is what is making everyone balloon. For years, we've been told that fat is to blame, which ended up with products being stripped of their fat content and labelled 'diet' or 'light'. Diet product, me hole. When the manufacturers removed the fat, this removed the flavour along with it, so then they just pumped their products full of sugar instead. Pricks. Well, at least our videos were getting the message out there. In addition, it was a landmark moment for me as for the first time ever, when I saw myself on screen, I was happy with how I looked. I had nothing to criticise. I was slim, I looked ten years younger than my age, and I could see the change in the shape of my body since training with weights. I looked really well and for the very first time, watching myself in a video, I could accept that. So that was huge, and I was small. And shockingly, Siobhan was silent.

When the one-year anniversary of my surgery rolled around, I decided to celebrate by dressing up as J-Lo for Hallowe'en. This was the first year ever that I could wear a sexy costume, so I thought, 'Tonight, Matthew, I'm going to be Jennifer Lopez.' You know her iconic green tropical print dress with the big split up the leg and down the front that made her famous? Yeah, well that's Versace, so I couldn't afford it, so I went on eBay and got a 20 quid version, a catsuit in the same tropical print like the one she wore in her 'Hey Papi' music video. Jaysus, she's such a lash bag. Gold lamé bra, big hoop earrings and aviators on, I rocked out that night, thanking Matt for making me do so many squats in the gym. My ass wasn't of quite J-Lo proportions, but for a bird with Irish DNA I was looking good. Hardly a professional J-Lo lookalike, now, but I felt fab. My new rule with myself these days is that I make an effort with my clothes seven days a week. If I'm not in Lycra gym gear, I'm in mini-skirts, skinny jeans, tight tops or fitted dresses and that's just during the day. I spent so long camouflaged in my black uniform so now I've broken out of fat prison, I wear sexy clothes because I finally can and it feels incredible. The scars on my tummy are practically invisible and I can now wear a bikini with confidence. My body is not perfect, but it is good enough.

Since I started dressing like a ride, I noticed men checking me out everywhere I went. I hadn't experienced this for so long, and it felt fantastic. Before, when I'd walk down the street, I may as well have been invisible (because that's what I needed to be mirrored back to me), but now I was getting wolf whistles from builders and mechanics and in general loads of men were staring as I'd teeter past in my micro miniskirts. I was convinced that as soon as I became slim, I'd be beating the guys off with a stick and would easily bag myself a boyfriend. But did any of these stare-bears chat me up on a night out? That would be a no. Twelve months on as a size 10 and in that time do you know how many dates I've been on? One. And of course, being the Bridget Jones that I am, I royally fecked that up. I'm 36 years old, but it was like sending the 18-year-old me on the date because I was so out of practice and hadn't a rashers what to do. Sure I'd never really been on a date before. Even back when I was 18, I wasn't going on proper dates with guys, I was only a kid. The problem I have is that if I fancy a man, I can't talk to him. I just clam up and can't be myself. I've thought a lot about why I do this and I think it's because I know I like him and I'm afraid that if I show my true self to him and he rejects me, then I'll be devastated. If I don't reveal myself, then I can't get hurt. Does that make sense? The explanation, I mean, not the action, because I know that doesn't make sense. What a stupid feckin' thing to do! I know, but I can't help it. It just consumes me and happens without my permission. And it's not Siobhan's fault. It's like a natural body and mind instinct that seizes me.

The one date was with a guy I knew, not very well or anything, but I hadn't seen him for a good ten years. We bumped into each other on a night out and ended up snogging. And then texting. I'm brilliant on the texts, I can dish out the witty banter like there's no tomorrow, but in the flesh I just can't fully be myself. I go mute because my brain seems to rewire itself and I can't think of anything witty or intelligent to say. So when he invited me to his place for dinner, I had to down a large vodka before I headed over there to try and calm my nerves. At this point in my journey I was 11 stone and I looked great, but I was still smack in the middle of the mind-melt, with my brain trying to catch up with my body and remember that I wasn't big anymore. So on the date, predictably enough, I struggled to be myself. I was so self-conscious and the whole time Siobhan was telling me, 'There's no way he could fancy you. Like, fancy you? What's to fancy? This must be a wind-up. I guarantee he's only on this date for a bet. Where are the hidden cameras?'

Surprisingly, the first date led to a second date, purely, I think, because I was able to redeem myself via post-date amusing text messages that sold me in a better light. I made him dinner at my place and the nerves and Siobhan's berating led to me drinking copious glasses of wine. I ended up a drunken eejit, sliced my finger open on the foil of the wine bottle and served up the dinner with a blood-drenched hand. Later I tried to sit down on the sofa but missed it and fell off it onto the floor and God only knows what else I did or said as drunken Siobhan puppeteered my bodily functions and I made a right twat of myself. Needless to say, that was the end of that and he avoided me thereafter while I continued to send him drunken texts for months. Oh Jules, you absolute tool. I know, I know. But I've deleted and blocked his number and email now so Siobhan has absolutely zero ways of contacting him, no matter how pissed she is. Phew!

At 36 I have to admit I have heard my ovaries ticking for quite some time now. I would love to have a husband and kids someday soon. But how am I supposed to do that when I can't get chatted up, let alone go on another date that I could attempt to try and be myself on? Yes, I've been on all the dating websites and they make me feel even more disheartened and I've done speed-dating as well, again with no luck. Yet again, hello mirrors. Nobody was hitting on me when I was overweight because I believed I was unattractive and not worthy of being chatted up, so why weren't men chatting me up now that I had accepted myself as being attractive and felt so much better in myself being slim? The answer I found was that I needed to work on falling in love with myself instead of depending on a man to fall in love with me and give me those feelings of love. I needed to have them 100% for myself and from myself, so then he can step in and reflect that love back to me. As they say, you shouldn't need another half to complete you. You should feel whole in yourself and then have a partner that you can share your love, life and experiences with. So loving myself in an all-encompassing way is a project I've been working on for the past few months. I don't know how long it's going to take, but by Jaysus I'm trying.

Siobhan keeps asking me, 'You can't get a boyfriend. What is wrong with you?' I have put that question to men on nights out and the reply I've received from several of them is that apparently I'm quite intimidating and they wouldn't come near me in a million years. For feck's sake. Me, intimidating? Just because I'm wearing a sexy dress? I don't rock around like a peacock who's unapproachable. Hang on, mirrors, Jules, mirrors! They think I'm intimidating, what's the reflection? I'm intimidated by men I fancy. Aaaah! That's it! Right, that's what I need to heal. I just worked that out now. The mirrors are feckin' great, aren't they? Initially, I thought maybe I should tone down the sexy dresses and make myself more 'girl next door' so men would find it easier to approach me on a night out and then I thought, 'You know what, feck that, I won't.' I'm not going to water myself down because he can't handle me at 100-proof. I'm enjoying my new sexy look and if a fella doesn't have big enough balls to approach me, then he's not the fella for me. I need a guy with bowling balls who'd look at me and say, 'Yeah, I'm gonna try my luck!' As it happens, that big-balled boy did just that on New Year's Eve, 31 December 2015.

Wearing a very short tartan mini-skirt (something I'd always dreamed of wearing after seeing it on Rachel in *Friends*), I strolled through Dunnes Stores, having bought some booze for my lonely night in by myself, ringing in the new year. I couldn't be arsed going out as the countdown was always shite, mainly because I never had anybody to kiss at midnight. As I stood beside my car rooting in my bag for my keys, I was approached by a handsome guy who nervously introduced himself as Dave and asked me if I'd like to go for a coffee with him sometime. I was so startled I went Pikachu puce and I remember putting my hands up to my face like a giggling Japanese school girl who'd just met a life-size Hello Kitty. I just said, 'Sorry, what?!' and he repeated his introduction. I was so shocked that someone was chatting me up, but not only that, it was in the middle of the day in a car park! A man with balls! Balls of steel! I was so impressed. He was nervous and I knew by him that he didn't do this on a regular basis. He told me he had seen me walking past and was compelled to come over and talk to me. 'Marry me, you absolute ride!' I thought in my head. Instead, I told him how cool I thought it was that'd he chat me up in the middle of the afternoon in a supermarket car park. He was handsome and refined, so I said I'd love to go for coffee with him and he could have my number. He was delighted and whipped out his phone. I called out my number and with the nerves he realised he was typing it into his phone calculator instead of contacts. We laughed about that and I called it out again. We chit-chatted for a minute and then off he went.

I was shaking as I rang my best friend Donna and told her the news. 'Teddy! Oh my God! A guy just chatted me up and asked me out on a coffee date! A man, Teddy! A real man! I can't flippin' believe it!' I screeched down the phone. Donna was beside herself with glee for me and was shrieking back just as loudly. Only your best mate can appreciate moments like this, especially as she's seen me eternally single. Of course, within minutes we were planning the wedding. 'What a way to end 2015,' I thought. Hello 2016. I couldn't wait for him to call!

Three dismal weeks passed and not a sausage. I was so surprised, considering the definite attraction when we'd first met. Of course I went full Angela Lansbury on the net, trying to track him down, but with such little information to go on, not even my top-notch online stalking skills could come up with a lead. Listening to my intuition, which always guides me in the right direction, I decided to email me aul pal Ray D'Arcy as he has played detective in situations like this before and managed to hunt down people via his radio show appeals. So I lobbed off an email to Ray explaining my predicament and that I was sure Dave had taken down my number wrong. All I had to go on was his first name, where the chatting up took place and that I think he had said he was from Killiney in South Dublin. Ray invited me into the RTÉ radio station the following day and we had a chat on air. The texts started pouring in, with most saying, 'He's a married man who was just chatting her up to see if he could get her number and tell himself that he's still got it.' What? He was not married. I was there, I knew by him. His nerves were endearing and this

349

was genuinely a lovely guy chatting me up. Cryin' out loud, Ireland! Where's the positivity? Sadly, the appeal garnered no leads as the now nicknamed Dunnes Dave never came forward.

Like loads of girls in Ireland, I've had a crush on Ray D'Arcy since he was on *The Den*, so when he invited me to be a guest on his Saturday night TV show I jumped at the chance. The plan was to have the chats about life since *Nine Stone Lighter*, the book deal I'd just signed, my new fit life and my videos about the dangers of sugar that went viral. As I sat in the green room beforehand with Donna, Ray came over to say hello and I told him how much I was looking forward to the interview. Ray then said, 'So we'll start with Dave and end with Dave.' I froze. Speechless. I didn't know that Dunnes Dave was going to be discussed?! I didn't say a word because I thought that Ray might have put his foot in it and accidentally revealed that Dave was in fact here in the building and they were going to bring him out and surprise me. As soon as Ray walked away from the table, Donna and I turned and looked at each other and at the same time said, 'He's here!' I nearly vommed. I wasn't at all prepared for this and it was a total curve ball when the interview was all about Dunnes Dave and I was bricking it that I was coming across as a desperado trying to track down a random man I knew nothing about who had chatted me up for all of three minutes in a supermarket car park. Through the course of the conversation I also ended up admitting to Ray, and the 400,000 people watching the show, that I'd never had a boyfriend. How fucking embarrassing. Sigh. And no, Dave didn't appear out from backstage to surprise me. I got that all wrong. I truly am Ireland's Bridget Jones. FMLL. In the following weeks, everywhere I went people would come up to me and ask, 'Did you find yer man Dunnes Dave?!' I would just cringe and tell them, 'No, no, I didn't.'

But little did I know that Dunnes Dave was actually watching the show. Nearly three months have passed since my appearance and yesterday I kept seeing posts on Facebook about a 'secret inbox of Facebook messages' we all have where spam is filtered. I've known about this extra inbox for years and I wondered why everyone was only finding out about it now. My whole newsfeed was full of posts about it, but I just scrolled past them. When Donna's boyfriend, Mark, mentioned it to me, I wondered why it was coming into my awareness yet again. So last night, while crashed out on my bed, cream-crackered after a 12-hour session of writing this book, I decided to have a look in my mystical secret inbox to see what messages were in it. I hadn't checked it for years and of course it was jam-packed with requests from the King of Tikkibutu telling me about how he wanted to transfer monies into my bank account to save his impoverished nation. Lo and behold, amongst all the spammage, who else was there a message from? Dunnes Dave!

> Hi Jules, it's Dave here. I just saw you on *The Ray D'Arcy Show* from last night. I must have taken down your number wrong because I sent a message and got no reply. It's great to be able to talk to you because I thought the number you gave me might have been fake but now I realise it wasn't. When I heard nothing from you I presumed you may not have been interested which is understandable, so I let it be. Consequently, I have been introduced to a girl by my friend who set me up recently. I think you would understand that it would be unfair on her not to give it a fair chance. It was great hearing about how exciting your life has been and will be, especially with the new book on the horizon. I hope this message finds you well and wish you all the best. Dave.

Isn't that gas? So he did take down the wrong number! (Note to self: in future, get him to dial the number on the spot to make sure he took it down correctly.) And he wasn't married and trying his luck to see if he still 'had it'. I knew it! That was the biggest relief of all because thinking that I was the piece of meat a married man would test out his levels of mojo on made me feel like crap. I replied to Dave, of course, and explained things from my end and wished him luck in his new relationship. I think he came into my path that day to give me the validation I needed that a man could find me attractive and chat me up. Okay, so nothing came of it, but thanks, Dunnes Dave, for giving me that boost of confidence that I needed. But how uncanny that I discovered that message from him, which he sent three months ago, on the day that I wrote about him in this book. There's a prime example of the law of attraction in action.

I have to say, it's so shite being forever single. I would love to have a boyfriend. I like to tell myself that I'm not actually single, I'm in a long-distance relationship because my boyfriend lives in the future. Sometimes I wonder if my standards are too high. I know what I want. Basically Mr Darcy from *Pride and Prejudice* ejaculating chocolate. Is that too much to ask? I also know what I don't want and that's the Milk Tray Man. If he crept in my balcony window and left a box of chocolates on my bedside table, I'd have to fling them back at him and say, 'There's about 60 teaspoons of sugar in that box! Get out, ya lunatic!' It really pisses me off when I see people in relationships and marriages and they take it for granted or else just don't bother putting the effort in. And their sex life decimates and they don't appreciate the fact that they have someone who loves them. To address it, we even wrote a scene about it in *Damo & Ivor* where a single Grano, who was desperate to find a man for herself, gets irate with Tracey, who doesn't appreciate her relationship with her boyfriend, Spuddy.

Grano: Jaysus, girls, St Anthony's after comin' up trumps again! The little lemon car broke down this mornin' and there I was standin' on da side of da road when I met this hunk of a fella. I'm not jokin', he's an absolute dreamboat! And wait'll ya hear this, girls, he wants to bring me out on a date this afternoon!

Tracey: And are ya goin'?

Grano (holding up shopping bag): Will ya stop, sure look! I'm just after clearin' out Ann Summers! Oh God, I tell ya it'll be great to get back up on the pogo stick!

Tracey: Jesus, I couldn't think of anything worse.

Grano: Wha'?! When was the last time you rode Spuddy?

Tracey: I dunno. Months ago.

Grano: You know what, that kinda thing really pisses me off. There ya are with sex on tap and you're probably givin' it the whole 'I've had a long day, I'm tired, I've got a headache' while us single ones couldn't get a ride off a bike! Poor Spuddy and you have him workin' around da clock he probably doesn't even have the time to give himself a hand shandy. I've a good mind to go over and give him rattle meself. The poor chap. Do you not love him?

Tracey: I do love him! I love him to bits!

Grano: Well, then get your arse home and show him!

Well, I tell ya, it'll be a lucky man who marries me because there'll be no pretend headaches when I'm around. I can't wait to meet him and for us to fall in love. I've got 20 years of shagging to make up for, so the poor chap is going to be on a Lucozade drip 24 hours a day and his willy is going to be in flithers. I'll have it whittled down from a totem pole to a cocktail stick in no time. God help him! He'll need to have the stamina of an Olympian to keep up with me in the sack. What a lucky fella. I'm dream girlfriend material. I only order a starter when out for dinner and two glasses of wine has me pissed. I'll always be up for the ride so I'm a cheap date by all accounts. It's gas to think that he's out there somewhere right now and has no idea what he's in for once our paths cross. I bet he'll have a ring on my finger by the end of the first date.

Hopefully my protein shake will bring all the boys to the yard and I know my Mr Right is out there somewhere and I'm sure we'll find each other someday soon. My intuition keeps telling me that as soon as I complete writing this book, as it's such a cathartic experience, he'll just waltz into my life and sweep me off my ten-stone feet. In fact, I'm sure of it. I know I will manifest my fairy-tale and, bunion or no bunion, I will fit my foot into that glass slipper! And my handsome prince and I will get married and I'll get into a size 10 wedding dress and be a ridey bride. Then I'll get pregnant and spit the baby out because my core muscles will be so strong from all the training with Matt. And I'll be a smug mum and get a 'baby on board' sticker for my car so other drivers can drive behind me and think, 'Oh, you have a baby on board? I'll just run into the car next to you instead.' And I will be the best wife ever because I will appreciate the relationship like nobody ever has before and he will treat me like I'm some sort of majestic endangered species that needs to be treasured. And we will raise the kids and send them to a non-denominational mixed school so they can mingle with the opposite sex and then we'll grow older and I'll go through the menopause, I've defeated the hormones once, so I'm sure I can do it again. And my life will continue to be a series of twists and turns and things to learn until my dying day. Because I now realise that happiness is not a destination, it's a state of being. Happiness doesn't depend on external circumstances because happiness is a choice. It's just a thought away.

I have now officially exited the Flabyrinth. And I'm happy to report that Siobhan and I have actually bonded. I've discovered that the voice is my head is in fact my ego filling my mind with spam. Siobhan is a false sense of identity that feels that she is not enough. I asked Siobhan, 'Is it true that I am worthless?' and when she couldn't answer to prove that I was, I knew it was time for me to stop believing the shite that she fed me. Now Siobhan can dissolve and I am free to be my authentic self. I am just Jules and I am 'flawsome' – an individual who embraces her flaws and knows that she is awesome regardless. This life is not a rehearsal, so I will continue to strive to live my best life, consistently making healthy choices and always aiming for 'good enough' because I am a work-in-progress and I always will be.

Fin.

# Want more?

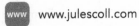 www.julescoll.com

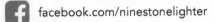 facebook.com/ninestonelighter

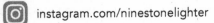 instagram.com/ninestonelighter

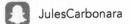 JulesCarbonara

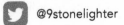 @9stonelighter